THE INFLUENCE OF
INDIVIDUAL DIFFERENCES
IN HEALTH AND ILLNESS

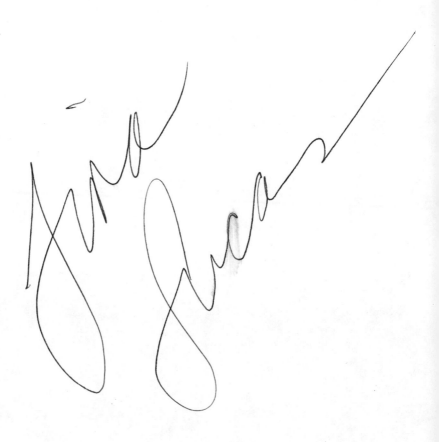

BEHAVIORAL SCIENCES
FOR HEALTH CARE PROFESSIONALS

Michael A. Counte, Series Editor

During the 1970s there was a rapid growth in the amount of behavioral science instruction included in the training of physicians, nurses, dentists, pharmacists, and other health care professionals. New faculty members were put on staffs at medical centers, curricula were devised, and on occasion new departments were created to support a diverse group of behavioral scientists.

The new emphasis on behavioral science in the education of health care professionals and the inclusion of a behavioral science section in certification examinations have generated a need for clinically relevant text materials. This series responds to that need by providing general, yet concise, introductions to common topical areas in behavioral science curricula, linking concepts and theories to clinical practice.

The authors of the series volumes are behavioral scientists with considerable experience in the education of health care professionals. Most of them are also clinicians, and their varied experience enables them to present their topics in a readable fashion. The content of the texts presumes only a very basic knowledge of the behavioral sciences, and emphasis is placed on the practical implications of research findings for health care delivery.

It is our hope that this multivolume approach will allow each instructor to select the books most pertinent to his or her particular curriculum. The division of topics was planned to enhance the overall flexibility of the information being presented.

Titles in This Series

Also of Interest

† Available in hardcover and paperback.

THE INFLUENCE OF INDIVIDUAL DIFFERENCES IN HEALTH AND ILLNESS

Linas A. Bieliauskas, Ph.D.

Rush-Presbyterian-St. Luke's Medical Center

The notion of individual differences in health and illness stems from the unique organization of behavior that profoundly affects how each individual maintains health, expresses and experiences symptoms of illness, and reacts to efforts at treatment. It is difficult to fully understand the interaction between personality and physical well-being because there is no universally accepted explanation of *why* we behave as we do; nor do we have any one theory that can unfailingly predict *what* we will do in every situation. Instead, health care professionals are faced with a dazzling array of theories, each of which has its own merits and makes its own contribution to unraveling the mysteries of individual differences in health and illness.

Dr. Bieliauskas provides a basic, concise introduction to theories of personality and other concepts of behavioral organization for those who have not had extensive coursework in the behavioral sciences. His aim is to help health care professionals begin to recognize patterns of behavior and to make it easier for them to understand and interpret comments offered by mental health consultants in the health care setting. For those who wish to read further, Dr. Bieliauskas also provides an extensive bibliography.

Dr. Linas A. Bieliauskas is director of clinical training and assistant professor of psychology at Rush-Presbyterian-St. Luke's Medical Center in Chicago. He is the author of another book in this series, *Stress and Its Relationship to Health and Illness* (1981).

To my parents,
Vytautas J. Bieliauskas, Ph.D., and Danute G. Bieliauskas, M.D.

BEHAVIORAL SCIENCES FOR HEALTH CARE PROFESSIONALS

THE INFLUENCE OF INDIVIDUAL DIFFERENCES IN HEALTH AND ILLNESS

Linas A. Bieliauskas, Ph.D.

Rush-Presbyterian-St. Luke's Medical Center

Westview Press / Boulder, Colorado

Behavioral Sciences for Health Care Professionals

Copyright © 1983 by Westview Press, Inc.

Published in 1983 in the United States of America by
Westview Press, Inc.
5500 Central Avenue
Boulder, Colorado 80301
Frederick A. Praeger, President and Publisher

Library of Congress Cataloging in Publication Data
Bieliauskas, Linas A.
  The influence of individual differences in health and illness.
  (Behavioral sciences for health care professionals)
  Bibliography: p.
  Includes index.
  1. Medicine and psychology. 2. Individuality. 3. Personality. I. Title. II. Series.
R726.5.B53   1983   150'.24616   82-13461
ISBN 0-86531-004-1
ISBN 0-86531-005-X (pbk.)

Printed and bound in the United States of America

CONTENTS

TABLES AND FIGURES

1

THE NOTION OF INDIVIDUAL DIFFERENCES

The concept of individual differences reflects the idea that while there may be abilities and characteristics common to all persons, there is a distinct uniqueness to each of us that accounts for a significant proportion of behavioral variation. This uniqueness makes it difficult to rely on general rules or principles for understanding the behaviors we see in an individual. In a medical context, it makes it hard to make sense out of complaints, symptoms, and reactions of specific patients. Some people who are basically in good health can exhibit marked concerns about their well-being or even show symptoms that are consistent with serious illness. Others with significant physical disease may have few symptoms and pay little attention to their deteriorating state of health. Weinman (1981) breaks down these differences between patients into five areas: (1) symptom perception, or the way that bodily changes (such as pain) are perceived and labeled by individuals; (2) symptom action, or what a person does in response to the perception of a symptom (such as seeking medical attention); (3) symptom formation, that is, the differential proneness of people to various disorders (for example, the increased risk of heart disease associated with the "Type A" personality described in Chapter 8); (4) response to illness, or adjusting to the demands illness places on a person's life; and (5) response to treatment, such as communication with medical personnel, tolerance to medications, and so on. In this volume, we will be concerned with increasing the understanding of the unique organization of behavior in each of us and how that pattern relates to health and illness.

1

For some theorists, uniqueness determines behavior to such a degree that individuals are seen as living primarily according to their own views of the world, which may have little basis in reality (Vaihinger, 1925). It is not what in reality happens to a person or the situation or surroundings in which a person exists that influences behavior, but rather the person's subjective appraisal of all these factors through the window of the "fictional" ideas (beliefs about reality) that govern his or her life. For example, someone who believes "honesty is the best policy" will make a drastically different response to an incident, such as reporting an automobile accident to an insurance company, than someone who espouses "look out for number one." Alfred Adler (1930), regarded as the father of individual psychology, expanded this concept of fictional ideas to the principle of "fictional finalism" – individual behavior is governed by unique personal goals that may have little to do with reality.

Concentrating on the individuality of the person is known as the "idiographic" approach to the study of behavior, a term coined by another champion of individual psychology, Gordon Allport (1962). The alternative approach is to concentrate on commonalities of behavior – the "nomothetic" approach. Allport argued strongly for the individual approach because he believed that most research on behavior had blurred the qualities of the individual by submerging them within universal laws and general variables. He further believed that individual qualities are the primary determinants of behavior and that neglect of these qualities leads to an ineffective understanding of behavior.

Let us take a preliminary look at how individual characteristics of behavior can have an impact on health-related difficulties. Consider two individuals who, because they live in a poor section of a city, belong to a low socioeconomic group, and are members of an ethnic minority, would be considered at high risk for a variety of illnesses such as cancer, heart disease, and viral infection. These individuals would also be likely to engage in behaviors, such as increased alcohol consumption, increased smoking, and poor eating habits, that contribute to an increased risk for a variety of diseases. One of the two individuals we are considering might refrain from alcohol, drugs, or smoking because of fundamental religious beliefs that have shaped his view of the world in such a way that he sees these behaviors as evil and therefore incongruent with his goal of "being holy." The other individual also refrains from such behaviors, but he does so because he views himself as the leader of a peer group in which he must maintain his wit and strength to keep his position secure. These individuals would both avoid the increased health risk associated with the above-mentioned behaviors, but for entirely different reasons. Their two distinct personalities, organized in different ways, both contribute to the same result in terms of health.

Now, let us consider the same two individuals hospitalized following an automobile accident. The first individual might view the accident as an act of God that carries a message for him. In the hospital, he might see the attending personnel as being part of a divine plan and put his faith in that plan to take care of him. In a practical sense, he would probably be compliant with medical procedures and would tend to obtain maximum benefit from his hospital stay. The second individual may see his hospitalization as a threat to his leadership status, since it has taken him away from his peer group, and he may object to the generally dependent role forced on him as a patient—a role at considerable variance with his self-image and goals. He is far less likely to do well during his hospital stay in terms of compliance with medical procedures and taking advantage of a necessary rest. Nevertheless, the effectiveness of his treatment could be improved if his individual characteristics were taken into consideration; medical personnel could encourage his friends or family to reassure him about his status and he could be given some sense of control over and participation in his treatment plan.

So, although both of our hypothetical individuals are members of the same sociocultural group with the same risks of disease as others in their situation, individual factors modifying high-risk behaviors may prevent either of them from becoming ill. However, if an accident were to occur to each of them, they might for the same reasons react quite differently to treatment, with significant consequences for recovery of health. The differences between these two individuals are significant determinants of their behavior in comparison to more general influences on health and illness.

The way in which behaviors are uniquely organized in each individual can be called that individual's "personality." Allport (1937, p. 48) defined personality as "the dynamic organization within the individual of those psycho-physical systems that determine his unique adjustment to his environment." He later altered the latter part of this definition to substitute "determine his characteristic behavior and thought" (Allport, 1961). This characteristic behavior and thought is not only different between individuals, it also is likely to have formed in different ways, for different reasons.

Let us again consider our two hypothetical individuals. The one with the predominantly religious orientation might have an unconscious identification with his church that replaces a lost or nonexistent relationship with his father. Through family interaction, he may have learned at an early age that to be accepted and protected he needed to live in a way that was regarded as "good"; thus he has always behaved like a "good boy." From a learning standpoint, it is likely that he received rewards both within and outside his family for behavior consistent with this image; the rewards might have included praise, respect, or possible protection from danger. This individual's view of the world is solidly structured in terms of good and evil, right and wrong; it would be difficult for him to change that viewpoint if circumstances changed and it became inefficient. In addition to these factors our individual might also have specific attributes tailored to the overall organization of his personality. He might have a general ability to do things that is effective in a structured, guided situation but not flexible or resourceful enough to deal with situations involving ambiguity or complexity. He may also have an externalized way of looking at the world around him – that is, seeing life events as not under his control. This view would be perfectly compatible with his system of rules and dogma concerning behavior.

The other individual we have been discussing, the group leader, would be quite different when viewed along the same dimensions. He might have a strong, unconscious identification with his father and strive to be like him. His father may have been a leader in his community, and the son may have expectations of leadership that were communicated to him since early childhood. He may have learned that the exercise of power was usually rewarded – for example, through respect, prerogatives, and status. His resulting view of the world would be structured in terms of friends versus enemies, weak versus strong, and dangerous versus safe. His general ability to do things would probably be greater than that of his peers, thus permitting him to adapt to novel situations with an alacrity respected by others. He may have an internalized way of looking at the world – that is, he perceives what happens in his life as generally under his control.

As you can see, there are many different ways of looking at how behavior is organized in different persons. Unfortunately, there is no current, single, accepted theory of behavior that accounts for all the possibilities. Each of the many different theories of personality has its own merits, although no one theory can fully explain all aspects of behavior. Therefore, we will study a number of personality theories and individual concepts in an attempt to obtain an overall understanding of what guides human behavior. The next four chapters will focus on four major approaches to understanding individual personality, describing how these approaches would view difficulties associated with illness or behaviors conducive to health. The next two chapters will look at other factors regarded as important sources of differences in behavior between individuals and examine how they relate to health and illness. I will then provide an introduction to common methods of assessing individual differences, to be followed by a final chapter that attempts to integrate the various viewpoints in order to facilitate their application to the practice of health care. Our overall purpose is to explore those unique, idiographic aspects of behavior that provide the constant exceptions to the rules we usually apply when faced with an individual patient.

ANALYTIC APPROACHES

Taking an analytic approach to personality simply means that the organization of behavior is viewed as being made up of different parts. In this chapter, we will look at the theories of Sigmund Freud and Carl Jung as some of the best regarded attempts to view personality in this way. But before we look at these theories in more detail, it is important to understand that they are based on what is termed a "dynamic" perspective. This perspective assumes that behavior is governed by an impelling force or energy. Sullivan (1953, p. 103) defined the concept of a "dynamism" as "a relatively enduring pattern of energy transformation which recurrently characterizes the organism in its duration as a living organism." In Sullivan's opinion, behavior thus reflects the transformation of energy that emerges from certain sources.

Now, it should be kept in mind that the early dynamic theorists, while sometimes viewing this energy transformation as physically based, used the approach primarily as a conceptual vehicle. Once we have accepted the dynamic viewpoint as a model for understanding human behavior, we can then entertain the frameworks presented by these theorists without worrying too much about the plethora of terms, assumptions, and schemata that characterize them. It is necessary to include these frameworks in our study of personality because there is no current theory that can account for all human behavior, and the insights provided in each approach are therefore of considerable value when we are faced with the task of comprehending the behavior of the individual person.

In this chapter, I have kept the number of new terms to a minimum and limited the discussion of each theoretical perspective to a depth that is readily understandable. The reader who wishes to study these complex approaches in greater depth should refer to core texts in personality (e.g., Hall and Lindzey, 1970; Levy, 1970; Rychlak, 1973) and to the theorists' original works (Freud, 1953–1964; Jung, 1953–1971).

FREUD: PSYCHOANALYSIS

From a rather oversimplified standpoint, the theory of Sigmund Freud can be said to have conceptualized human behavior as resulting from a shifting of energy in a topographical field. In other words, behavior is the result of various factors impinging on a finite force within the boundaries of a defined map. Certain rules govern the way in which this force interacts with the factors affecting it and the pattern it follows on the map. These rules have certain broad definitions, although for the most part they are individually determined. The process of deciphering the organization of these rules in a given person is termed *psychoanalysis.* Let us examine the various components of the psychoanalytic theory of personality.

Libido

The force, or psychic energy, that powers the personality is called the *libido;* it drives all behavior. Freud described the libido as "a quantitative magnitude . . . of the instincts which have to do with all that may be comprised under the word 'love'" (1961, p. 17). In his description, Freud placed a heavy emphasis on sexual desire as a basic impulse impelling the libido—that impulse being to seek pleasure and avoid pain. The libido, in following this impulse, thus operates according to the *pleasure principle.* Unfortunately, over the years, Freud's emphasis on sexuality has been overidentified with genital pleasure alone, rather than with the broader meaning of pleasure that he intended. Consequently, many people have come to regard the libido as a meaningless construct; it seems unlikely, after all, that prepubescent children could be genitally motivated or that the whole human race could be "sex-crazed." But Freud never intended these conclusions to be drawn; rather, he defined the sexual impulse as a pleasure-seeking impulse, including, but not limited to, genital pleasure. In this sense, according to Freud, one of the two basic impulses motivating human behavior is sexual.

The other basic impulse is aggression. Freud extended his description of the principal operation of the libido to include a "death instinct, an innate desire to return to the inorganic state" (Freud, 1955). He considered this instinct also to be in some sense a pleasure-seeking impulse consistent with the overall functioning of the libido. Since all living processes emanate from and eventually return to an inorganic state, the death instinct reflects a tendency to return to this earlier state, a state of ultimate quiescence (Rychlak, 1973). The impulse derived from this death instinct is aggression, a self-destructive tendency that, when frustrated, can be turned against others.

A further description of Freud's reasoning would fall beyond the scope of this text. It is sufficient to say that the arguments of Freud suggest that the two basic impulses governing human behavior are sexual and aggressive.

Developmental Theory

The developmental approaches of Freud and others are described in some detail in other volumes in this series (Billingham, 1982; Lopez and Feldman, 1982). For our purposes, I will make only brief mention of Freud's developmental schema, since it is germane to his conception of how the personality forms.

As mentioned above, the libido operates primarily in response to the sexual impulse. In the developing child, the libido seeks pleasure according to the various sensory foci (erogenous zones) to which the child of a given age attends. Thus, the first two years of a child's life are classified as *the oral stage* since pleasure is sought primarily through the mouth. The second stage, from approximately two to three years of age, is *the anal stage*. During this stage, parental demands center around toilet-training activities, and taboos over behavior are established. *The phallic stage*, from approximately three to six years of age, often involves touch and manipulation of sex organs. Pleasure can be obtained from this action, although not in the adult sexual sense. In addition, the child is acutely aware of similarities and differences between his or her sexual organs and those of the parents. *The latency stage,* from approximately age six to puberty, is the time when sex roles become defined through play and, as the name implies, is a quiet time in the child's life.

9

The final stage, *the genital stage,* begins with puberty and lasts throughout adulthood. Heterosexual attachments occur, and there is a shift of interest from self to others. As Hall and Lindzey (1970, p. 39) have noted, "In childhood, the sexual instincts are relatively independent of one another, but when the person reaches puberty they tend to fuse together and to serve jointly the aim of reproduction."

It is important for people to pass through these stages successfully. In each of these stages, the libido invests its energies in an action or an image that will gratify the sexual instinct associated with that stage. Thus, in the oral stage, the libido invests its energies (or, in psychoanalytic terms, forms a *cathexis*) in a particular object of relevance—namely, the mother, who is the source of food and stimulation for the oral area. The individual is highly dependent on others at this time. The successful passage through the oral stage requires that the strivings of the libido are not frustrated. If they are, then a fixation takes place; that is, the libido is trapped in an unfulfilled state and continues to exert an influence on personality as the individual matures, in a constant attempt to gratify its needs. An individual fixated at the oral stage is thus described as an oral personality, characterized by strong dependency needs and highly concerned with activities such as eating, drinking, smoking, or any other activity associated with the mouth. The same can be said for fixation at the other stages. The anal personality results from a frustration of pleasure associated with the anal zone, often caused by excessive conflicts during toilet training. Such a person tends to be orderly, controlling, and obstinate. The phallic personality tends to be flirtatious, egotistic, and promiscuous, resulting from frustration of pleasure sought through the sexual organs. The cathexis associated with these latter two stages may also be directed toward the parents and/or any other significant persons (and even objects) involved. It is also possible that frustration at each of these stages can be so intense that the libido seeks the avoidance of pain associated with the aggressive instinct, as opposed to the pursuit of pleasure associated with the sexual instinct; the avoidance of all unpleasant stimulation, the ultimate quiescence, may predominate. Because of the generally greater frustrations experienced by the individual during the anal stage, it is believed that anal personalities are generally aggressive. It is also for this reason that certain self-destructive tendencies are often associated with excessive dependency needs (frustration in the oral stage) or with abnormal patterns of sexual behavior (frustration in the phallic stage).

In summary, the libido is a form of psychic energy that operates according to sexual and aggressive impulses. These impulses are manifested differently depending on the stage of development and, through cathexes, leave lasting impressions on the organization of behavior.

The Topographical Map and the Unconscious

As mentioned earlier, the libido operates according to its impulses within a defined map. The map is composed of three areas: the *id*, the *ego*, and the *superego* (see Figure 1). The *id* constitutes the part of us that is basically instinctual. It operates primarily according to the pleasure principle and has no logic, morality, or consistency to its aims. As indicated in Figure 1, its content is entirely unconscious;

FIGURE 1. Freud's final mental structural constructs. (From Rychlak, 1981, Figure 4, p. 49. Reprinted by permission of Houghton Mifflin Company and the author.)

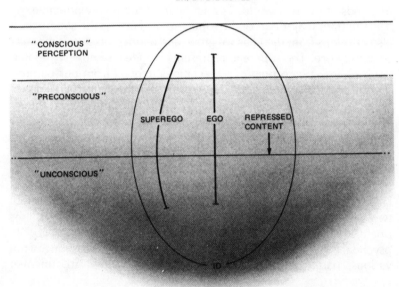

"EXTERNAL WORLD"

"CONSCIOUS" PERCEPTION

"PRECONSCIOUS"

SUPEREGO   EGO   REPRESSED CONTENT

"UNCONSCIOUS"

ID

Freud believed we can never fully know it. Yet, it is the source of the libido and thus exerts considerable influence over our behavior.

The ego is not present at birth; it develops out of the id as we grow and become aware of our surroundings. It is the part of us that is organized and that directs behavior. It functions in the service of the id in that it provides the reality contact necessary for the id to accomplish its goals. It thus operates according to *the reality principle*. As indicated in Figure 1, its content is primarily conscious, having been shaped by conscious factors; however, it also contains both unconscious and preconscious portions. The content of the unconscious portion, as in the id, is unknowable and instinctual. The preconscious portion is that "region of unawareness over which we often *do* have at least partial control" (Rychlak, 1973, p. 32). The preconscious is "made up of contributions from *both* the conscious and the unconscious, and it is the locus of censorship in the mind" (ibid., p. 32). Censorship is the act of preventing content from reaching consciousness because it is too threatening. This process of censorship is called *repression*. As seen in Figure 1, the process is in itself unconscious; that is, when we repress, we are not aware that we are repressing. For Freud, the unconscious therefore exerts considerable control over behavior, control we are often unaware of. The ego is the attempt to modify this influence according to the demands of the real world, as a function of the reality principle.

The third major part of the topographical map is the superego. It also develops from the id as we grow, and it functions as our morality or conscience. The superego represents the ideal of how we should behave, and it incorporates expectations derived from our parents, school, philosophy, religion, and so forth. It demands certain kinds of behavior of the ego and is frequently in direct opposition to the id. The superego thus acts according to what we might call *the morality principle*. Again, its content may be conscious or unconscious, and, as we can see in Figure 1, it has interactions with the id and ego on various levels to produce certain kinds of behaviors.

In sum, psychoanalytic theory takes the view that behavior is largely unconsciously determined and arises from the interaction of two primary impulses, the sexual and the aggressive. These impulses operate via the structure of the id, ego, and superego. In psychoanalysis, the ego is harnessed to explore the functioning of the various parts of this dynamic system in order to uncover preconscious content. This preconscious content provides clues about unconscious aspects of our behavior, thus leading to "insight" into what determines our actions.

Defense Mechanisms

When the individual is threatened by danger, the natural response is to become afraid. When the ego cannot bring fearful stimuli under control, *anxiety* is experienced. According to Hall and Lindzey (1970, p. 44):

> The function of anxiety is to warn the person of impending danger; it is a signal to the ego that unless appropriate measures are taken the danger may increase until the ego is overthrown. Anxiety is a state of tension; it is a drive like hunger or sex but instead of arising from internal tissue conditions it is produced originally by external causes. When anxiety is aroused it motivates the person to do something. He may flee from the threatening region, inhibit the dangerous impulse, or obey the voice of conscience.

Freud described three types of anxiety. *Realistic* anxiety is tension resulting from real-world dangers—for example, the fear of going into battle. The second type, *neurotic* anxiety, is basically a fear that the instincts will get out of control and that punishment will follow. Often, the instinctual impulse is unrecognized (since it is unconscious), and thus neurotic anxiety is experienced as not being a part of the self. The third type, *moral* anxiety, is basically a fear of the conscience, a feeling of impending guilt about doing something one shouldn't do. As you might guess, this type of anxiety is most prominent in individuals with a strongly developed superego.

Anxiety is a signal of threat that, as stated above, motivates the individual to do something about the threat. The individual deals with this threat by means of a *defense mechanism*.

Defense Mechanism

Repression:	Exclusion of specific thoughts, memories, impulses, feelings, and actions from awareness; motivated forgetting. This action is unconscious.
Suppression:	Motivated forgetting; but unlike repression, the action is conscious.

13

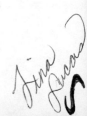

Reaction formation: Translation of repressed motives to their opposite; e.g., showing excessive affection and caring to a parent one intensely dislikes. This action is generally unconscious.

Denial: Reaction involving repression; refusal to accept or to recognize situations — instead, seeing things on an internal basis, e.g., being cheerful when faced with a life-threatening disease. This reaction is usually partially unconscious. *Defense Mech*

Displacement: Directing hostility or other feelings toward substitute objects or persons when the original object cannot be directly addressed; e.g., following reprimand by boss, taking frustrations out on one's family. This action is often partially unconscious.

Projection: Attributing one's unacknowledged faults or unacceptable motives to others, or assuming others possess the same traits and motives as oneself; e.g., the unscrupulous businessman who assumes that hospital personnel are out to swindle him. This action is generally unconscious. *Schizophrenia – Phobia, & Paranoid*

Sublimation: Satisfaction of socially unacceptable motives with socially acceptable behavior; e.g., the aggressive youngster who pursues a career in surgery. This action is at least partially unconscious.

Acting-out: Behavior that exhibits repressed motives, thus reducing anxiety; e.g., the teenager who indulges in promiscuous behavior as an outlet for aggressive motives toward parents. This action is usually partially unconscious.

These are only some of the many defense mechanisms that may serve to alleviate anxiety in the functioning personality. As you can see, certain obvious behaviors may have very subtle causes, which in themselves are difficult to discern without some understanding of the unconscious determinants of behavior.

JUNG: ANALYTICAL PSYCHOLOGY

In contrast to Freud, who viewed individuals as primarily driven by instinctual impulses, Carl Jung viewed personality as reflecting an historic as well as an individual past and a self-guided future. Although Jung likewise viewed the libido as a basic energy force, he further imbued it with a deterministic property—the capacity for making sense of experience. We can best understand Jung's view of personality by building on our discussion of the Freudian perspective.

The Principle of Opposites

Jung built his theory around the idea that each aspect of personality has a balanced counterstructure. For example, consciousness is balanced by the unconscious. Jung defined the ego as a comprehensive view of the self that the individual acknowledges and presents to others. The *shadow* is the hidden self, a portion of the personal unconscious known as the *alter ego*. It is the side of personality seen by the individual as distasteful or evil. (See Figure 2 for a partial representation of this personality organization.)

FIGURE 2. The psyche as personality. (From Rychlak, 1973, Figure 10, p. 142. Reprinted by permission of Houghton Mifflin Company and the author.)

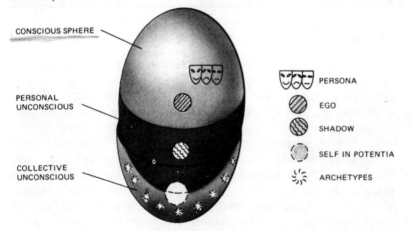

CONSCIOUS SPHERE

PERSONAL
UNCONSCIOUS

COLLECTIVE
UNCONSCIOUS

PERSONA

EGO

SHADOW

SELF IN POTENTIA

ARCHETYPES

Jung believed that the libido is generated by this differentiation into opposites. As psychic opposites are pulled into independent contents, psychic energy is turned loose. This concept of psychic energy, or libido, is thus expanded beyond Freud's notion of following a sexual instinct reflecting the strength of personal values or desires; the more value we invest in a particular kind of identification, the more the opposite of that identification is also formed and the more energy is released. For Jung, therefore, libido comes to mean something close to wanting or will.

The energy generated by such differentiation becomes available to form *complexes*. Jung sees all emotional reactions as stimulating mental thoughts that form groups of ideas or complexes; the strength and endurance of a complex is dependent upon the amount of emotion attached to it. In this context, Jung viewed the ego as an ego-complex; that is, the self-image is generated from the values tied to such concepts as "good," "smart," "hard worker," and so on. The shadow thus becomes the opposite complex, including qualities such as "bad," "unintelligent," and "lazy." The more libido freed in the formation of certain complexes, the more is available to form the opposites. This process can have a snowballing effect in which the individual appears to be taken over by another personality—as in the Dr. Jekyll–Mr. Hyde duality. This idea leads to the assumption that there is good and evil in each of us and offers a guide as to why certain kinds of behavior appear in a given person that are inconsistent with what we would expect.

The Collective Aspects of Personality

In addition to the personal aspects of consciousness and unconsciousness, Jung described the concept of collective aspects of personality—namely, the aspects we share with others. He specifically used the concept of the *persona* to describe a collective consciousness, the aspect of our behavior that we present directly to the world. The persona is analogous to a mask, what other people see. It is formed from societal restrictions, parental expectations, and so on; thus, it is not unlike Freud's concept of the superego. Jung suggested that the persona represents a certain danger because the individual may come to identify the persona as his or her real self rather than as the part of the self it truly represents. This process is sometimes seen to occur when famous figures in our society come to believe that their portrayals by the media represent the individuals they really are.

At the opposite end of the spectrum from the collective conscious is the collective unconscious—the system of beliefs, themes, and myths shared by all humans since the beginning of mankind. A single myth or belief is called an *archetype*. Archetypes in the collective unconscious might be ideas about a supreme being, immortality, hunting for food, and so on. According to Jung, these aspects of the unconscious are in each of us and, if given enough energy, may emerge into behavior. A good example of the emergence of archetypes into behavior would be the literary portrayal of the dog Buck in Jack London's *The Call of the Wild* (1960).

The Functions of the Psyche

Jung saw certain basic functions within the psyche as remaining constant relative to the changing conditions of life. There are four such functions, categorized as irrational and rational functions. *Sensation* is the first irrational function; it ascertains that something is there. The opposite irrational function is *intuition*; it ascertains where something came from and where it goes. *Thinking* is the first rational function and establishes what is there. *Feeling*, the opposite rational function, ascertains whether or not the individual wishes to accept what is there.

The ego generally identifies with one function in particular; this is termed the *superior* and *primary* function. The opposite function is the *inferior* function. The former governs the conscious way of interpreting reality, the latter the unconscious. The other two functions are *auxiliary* functions; one is *secondary* and conscious, whereas the opposite is unconscious. An individual can thus function primarily in a rational manner in terms of thinking and secondarily in an irrational manner in terms of sensation. Such an organization is depicted in Figure 3.

In sum, Jung differed from Freud in seeing beyond the basic instincts of sexuality and aggression as sole motivating forces in behavior, in accounting for the collective aspects of personality, in viewing the principle of opposites as the source of psychic energy, and in assigning functional styles to behavior. Of course, the theoretical differences are much greater than those presented here,

FIGURE 3. The four basic functions of the psyche. (From Rychlak, 1973, Figure 14, p. 164. Reprinted by permission of Houghton Mifflin Company and the author.)

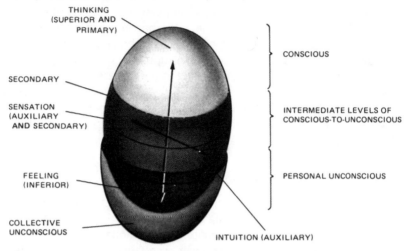

and the theories themselves are much more complex. These brief descriptions do, however, serve to introduce us to some basic conceptions of personality. If necessary, the reader is again referred to the basic texts mentioned earlier for a fuller understanding.

APPLICATIONS IN HEALTH AND ILLNESS

Both Freud and Jung emphasized that there are strong unconscious influences on behavior, influences that are not under obvious reality control. These approaches are not as popular today as they were twenty years ago, although they remain useful in determining the antecedents of an individual's behavior. Using the Freudian perspective, the health care professional may try to discover the basic sexual (pleasure-seeking) or aggressive (destructive) impulse underlying an individual's behavior. He or she may also try to understand the individual's reactions to present life situations in terms of Freudian psychodevelopmental processes. From a Jungian standpoint, it may be of value to assess the complexes under which the behavior appears to be organized and then to infer the opposing complexes that may actually be guiding the behavior.

In more direct terms, the individual patient's characteristics can be conceptualized from an analytic viewpoint according to the categories described by Weinman (1981) in the first chapter. Are the patient's symptoms perceived as personally significant from a standpoint other than the strictly medical? For example, a diagnosis of cancer can be seen as a reaffirmation of identification with a parent who died of cancer. If such an identification were thwarted due to parental rejection, the diagnosis may provide a libido cathexis for dependency needs, and efforts to engage the patient in ameliorative therapy may be foiled. On the other hand, the patient may have a complex that, unconsciously, includes the role of being ill. In this case, the individual's response to associated symptoms might prompt seeking of medical attention, but with an unconscious desire that the diagnosis be confirmed. Symptoms may be formed in such an individual to an exaggerated degree or with personal overconcern; moreover, if diagnostic tests are inconclusive, the patient may become angry with the medical personnel, who in turn may be confused by the patient's reaction. The patient might also respond to a diagnosed cancer with marked demands on family and personnel that serve to meet certain dependency needs beyond any required by the immediate illness itself. The above scenario is not as farfetched as one might imagine; indeed, it tends to occur with frustrating frequency.

Beyond these considerations, however, analytic theory has influenced medicine in two major areas. The first area of influence concerns the role of psychological factors in causing or aggravating disease. Alexander (1950) described specific psychological conflicts as being major contributors to the genesis of seven diseases—namely, peptic ulcer, ulcerative colitis, hyperthyroidism, regional enteritis, rheumatoid arthritis, essential hypertension, and bronchial asthma. Dunbar (1943) had earlier offered a broader interpretation of psychological contributions to disease, suggesting that certain personality types, rather than specific conflicts, correlated with certain diseases.

Let us consider only one medical condition here: peptic ulcer. Peptic ulcer generally involves visceral ulcerations, but the term covers a group of diseases, chronic and acute, that vary by type, history, and precise anatomical location. The difficulties involved in defining the disease itself are well explained by Weiner (1977). Alexander (1950) described patients with peptic ulcer as having strong

19

dependency conflicts formed during the oral stage of development. These unconscious dependency needs are frustrated during
adulthood, especially under stressful conditions, and lead to increased gastric secretion and motility, thus causing ulceration. Note
the association between oral conflict and digestive system-related
disease. Weiner, Thaler, Reiser, and Mirsky (1957), in a study of army
inductees, concluded that those with peptic ulcer showed evidence
of "major unresolved and persistent conflicts about dependency and
oral gratification" (p. 9) in conjunction with a high rate of gastric
secretion. More recently, Ackerman, Manaker, and Cohen (1981)
concluded that a recent emotional separation or loss may be
associated with the onset of peptic ulcer in at least a subgroup of patients; the relationship between this finding and dependency conflicts can be readily inferred. However, the evidence has not been
overwhelming in support of the etiological hypothesis. Weiner (1977)
noted that only one-half to one-third of all patients with peptic ulcer
are hypersecretors of gastric acid; how could it be said that
psychological factors affect the rest? In general, although theorists
continue to suggest that orally related dependency needs
predominate among such patients, there is little solid evidence that
they are significant factors in the etiology of peptic ulcer. Nevertheless, analytic theory has proved valuable, given its emphasis on
the role of psychological factors in disease, and even today continues
to bear fruit in research concerning, for instance, the relationship between the Type A personality and heart disease (see Chapter 8).
Weiner (1977) provides an excellent discussion of a number of
disease entities and the hypotheses relating them to specific
psychological conflicts.

The second major impact of analytic theory on medicine is the
hypothesis that psychological conflict can be symbolically transformed to mimic physical symptoms or to employ physical symptoms
for achieving certain ends. When a symbolic transformation takes
place, anxiety, instead of being directly experienced, is "converted"
into a physical symptom; this is called a conversion reaction, or conversion hysteria. Historically, conversion reactions referred to loss of
muscular functions, but, more recently, they have come to be
regarded as including pain and other bodily sensations (Ziegler, Imboden, and Meyer, 1960).

In brief, when an impulse becomes particularly threatening and
the libido is thwarted from fulfilling it toward an intended object, it

may be transformed symbolically into a somatic symptom. Such a transformation may occur in the case of a daughter who must care for an ill father whom she intensely dislikes. She feels the obligation to minister to his needs, yet loathes her task and is quite angry toward him for putting her in this position. She experiences a paralysis of her right arm, in the absence of any physical cause. Under psychoanalysis, her anger toward her father may be brought to light; the paralysis might then be revealed as a means of preventing her from hitting her father in fulfillment of an aggressive impulse.

Such dramatic cases are infrequently seen. Nevertheless, I recently saw a young woman patient who presented with constant movements of her legs, a condition previously diagnosed as symptomatic of multiple sclerosis. She underwent a thorough neurological examination at our medical center, but no evidence of disease was found. In the meantime, I discovered that the woman had a husband with multiple sclerosis and that she spent much of her time caring for him. Following a psychological evaluation in which it was determined that her symptoms fit the picture of a conversion reaction, she was referred for psychotherapy. During the course of therapy, an intense anger toward her husband was revealed, an anger that she could not express because her husband was ill. The symptoms provided some outlet for her hostility and also served to place her in the same dependent role as her husband, thus defusing some of the resentment she felt in caring for him. When the anger became obvious in psychotherapy and the woman developed ways to express it appropriately, her symptoms vanished.

More frequently, we see patients who have pain or vague complaints that are greatly exaggerated beyond any physical concomitants but clearly have some psychological purpose. Pain that serves to remove an individual from an unpleasant or demanding situation is a common example. Often, the symptom itself is less distressing than the real or imagined situation. And so the health care professional looks on in amazement as the patient resists being told that presenting symptoms indicate no serious medical illness; the patient appears to *prefer* a diagnosis of illness.

The general notion of behavior as directed by unconscious impulses thus provides valuable insight into the behavior of individuals. Whether or not we subscribe to analytical theory in particular, the conceptual framework yielded by this approach can help us to provide better patient care.

21

INTERPERSONAL
APPROACHES

The theories of Freud and Jung placed the primary determinants of behavior within the person, largely at an unconscious level. Even though psychological conflicts are often formed in interaction with others, the nature of the internal energy (libido) directs the formation and outward expression of behavior. Alfred Adler and Harry Stack Sullivan, among others, felt that such an approach ignored the social influences on formation of personality. Individuals exist, they argued, in an interpersonal context, and ignoring this fact is to ignore what makes us individuals.

For the interpersonal theorists, dynamic structures or maps became less important, as did the role of the unconscious in organizing the personality. There was a concomitant decrease in special terminology, a development the reader may appreciate. As mentioned in the previous chapter, I can only hope to provide a superficial acquaintance with the more prominent aspects of these theories. For a more detailed explication, core personality texts and the theorists' own works should be consulted (Adler, 1968; Sullivan, 1953, 1964).

ADLER: INDIVIDUAL PSYCHOLOGY

Alfred Adler did not believe that unconscious forces in the individual exerted mysterious, independent power over behavior. He generally denied the influence of instincts in motivating behavior, a view quite at variance with that of Freud. Although he did acknowledge that an unconscious portion of personality exists, he

23

treated it rather lightly and felt that both the conscious and unconscious portions of personality strive for the same ends; individuals
never act at cross purposes with themselves. Adler thus had a holistic
view of personality.

In line with the holistic viewpoint, the individual was seen as ef-
fecting his or her own direction to life. Adler viewed the individual as
having a purpose, a goal, an idea. This idea—a growing concept of
life, a way of looking at the world—is formed in one's early years.
Adler (1964, p. 7) called it "the style of life"; the popular term is "lifestyle." The ego was considered to be the personality as a whole.
Rychlak (1973) suggested that the ego, for Adler, represented the
conscious aspects of life, whereas the lifestyle was more general and
included what was unconscious. The unconscious was seen by Adler
to be primarily that about our lives that we do not understand.

Basic Concepts

As mentioned in the first chapter, Adler believed in the principle
of *fictional finalism* as a guiding rule for behavior. That is, individuals
behave according to certain expectations of the future, whether or
not those expectations have anything to do with reality. The lifestyle
is formed between the ages of about three and five and continues
into adulthood. Adler felt that an individual's earliest memories could
thus give a clue to understanding his or her lifestyle. An example of
such an idea, or lifestyle, would be the "bad boy." Such ideas are
termed prototypes, in that they give a shape to the lifestyle. With a
prototype of "bad boy," an individual would tend to be naughty, non-
conformist, and daring; he would behave "as if" the idea were true
and would expect others to treat him accordingly.

According to Adler, the primary motive in determining ideas or
lifestyles is a social one; individual personalities are determined by
social concerns that include, but are not limited to, "cooperation, interpersonal and social relations, identification with the group, empathy, and so forth" (Hall and Lindzey, 1970, p. 125). This motive
performs the role played by the primary sexual impulse in Freud's
theory. Adler believed that interactions with others in the areas of
social interest shape the individual's ideas.

The interactions with others are governed by certain principles.

Striving for superiority is one such principle, maintaining basically that each of us has a will to power, to perfection. This principle implies that we all have an impulse to be the best, to develop to our maximum, in the end to advance society. However, the particular ways in which we strive to be superior, and whether or not they are laudable or dysfunctional, depends on early experiences. For example, an individual might strive for superiority through intellect as opposed to physical accomplishments. On the other hand, the striving might be for social goals or purely for self-aggrandizement.

Because the striving for superiority is a basic impulse, each of us has a sensitivity to *inferiority*, a subjective feeling of weakness or disability. This feeling often leads us to engage in *compensation* for our real or imagined weaknesses. Compensation can become a means for improving our lives. The ideas of inferiority and compensation introduced by Adler have also been popularized. An example would be the "Napoleon complex," that is, the idea that because an individual is of small stature, as was Napoleon, he feels inferior and goes to great lengths to prove himself better than others, as by conquering Europe. The latter action, as you might guess, would be termed *overcompensation*, that is, going well beyond normal limits in making up for a felt sense of inferiority. Although Adler believed in the Freudian concept of repression, he subordinated it to the defense mechanisms of compensation and overcompensation; repression, for Adler, described the mental state of individuals who were pursuing lifestyles without understanding why.

The *creative self* was, for Adler, the prime determinant of personality structure. The creative self operates according to the principles already described and includes all of Adler's other concepts as subordinate to it, including the notion of lifestyle. Adler's primary hypothesis about the creative self was that the individual is master of his or her own fate. There are no unconscious demons who force actions upon us; rather, we guide our lives, creating our own personalities. This construct essentially lays responsibilty for our actions at our own feet and, in spite of external influences, eschews the placing of blame on others for our behavior. Psychotherapeutic approaches utilizing this perspective thus concentrate on teaching the patient to recognize his or her lifestyle and to reorient the creative self to achieve effective personal goals.

Developmental Theory

Some mention must be made of certain developmental concepts important in understanding Adler's contributions to personality theory. Adler introduced a concept that has become quite popular, the notion of behavioral effects of birth order. Adler felt that birth order influenced the lifestyle an individual eventually adopts. The first child is an extension of parental authority. The middle child is neither the eldest and most adept, nor the youngest and most loved; this child wants to outshine the older sibling, often exhibits ambitiousness and jealousy, and has much drive but less respect for authority. The last born is the baby of the family, tends to be pampered, and grows up expecting others to do things for him or her. The youngest child is seen as having some of the same characteristics as the only child, except that the latter often becomes more of an individualist.

Adler also proposed stages of development for the child, although they were more fluid than those of Freud. He considered proper parenting to be a relationship of social trust, in which the attitude toward the child is neither authoritarian nor smothering. He felt that the school years are particularly formative in that they cultivate social interest and influence the child's lifestyle, further noting that children who are failures in school often fail in life. He did not believe in grade tracking, skipping grades, or intelligence measurements because he felt that academic performance is socioeconomically determined for the most part and that labels of this sort may be a disservice to disadvantaged children. Adolescence, Adler felt, is primarily a time for dealing with occupational problems, not sexual problems as Freud would have suggested. He saw the main problem of adulthood to be one of harmonizing occupational and family goals and believed love to be a more important instinct than sex. He felt that, in marriage, each mate must be more interested in promoting the happiness of the other than in securing his or her own gratification. Many marriages break up, he felt, because the partners are more concerned with receiving than with giving.

In sum, Adler described the main problems of living as occupational, social, and sexual, and saw the development of the individual as a matter of devising different methods of dealing with these problems.

Individual Difference Types

Although Adler's emphasis on the uniqueness of the individual might appear to rule out any attempt to categorize people according to types, he did describe some lifestyles that people typically develop. I will mention a few here. In particular, there are two primary approaches to solving problems; (1) seek the solution directly and openly, as an optimist; (2) seek the solution by means of devious schemes and withdrawal, as a pessimist. The latter type of problem-solver could be classified as having an *inferiority complex*, that is, one who operates on the basic assumption that he or she is inferior (Adler, 1954).

Adler also described three types of children who are likely to overcompensate: (1) children with weak or imperfect organs; (2) children who are treated with severity and little affection; and (3) pampered children (Adler, 1930).

Of final interest are Adler's descriptions of four approaches to reality taken by the majority of individuals. The first is the *ruling approach*, telling others what to do. The second is the *getting approach*, always trying to get something. The third is the *avoiding approach*, "avoiding all challenge or responsibility" (Rychlak, 1973, p. 116). The fourth is the *socially useful approach*, caring and working for others (Ansbacher and Ansbacher, 1956).

Overall, Adler's approach to personality theory dramatically reduces the role of the unconscious in determining behavior and places the burden of responsibility on ourselves as individuals. The primary motives for behavior are social in nature and are enacted through principles associated with living according to the ideas, or lifestyles, that we establish early in our lives. These principles are basically related to a striving for superiority, for achievement of maximum development in ourselves and in our fellow human beings.

SULLIVAN: INTERPERSONAL THEORY

Like Adler, Harry Stack Sullivan believed that the individual cannot exist apart from society and that personality is by necessity influenced by interpersonal factors. Thus, Sullivan believed the interpersonal situation to be the unit of personality; personality itself is only a hypothetical construct describing the situation.

27

Basic Concepts

According to Sullivan, there are various processes that characterize interpersonal interactions. The first and most basic – the *dynamism* – was already discussed at the beginning of Chapter 2. To repeat, a dynamism is the relatively enduring pattern of energy transformation that characterizes the organism in its duration as a living organism. Sullivan's concept of energy, however, is different from that employed by Freud and Jung. Simply stated, for Sullivan "an energy transformation is any form of behavior" (Hall and Lindzey, 1970, p. 141) – in terms of the dynamism, any pattern of behavior that is identifiable, that endures, and that repeats itself over time.

Sullivan identified two basic types of dynamisms. In the first category are *zonal dynamisms,* that is, behaviors associated with physical activities such as getting food, engaging in sex, seeking drink, and so on. Such dynamisms satisfy the basic needs of the individual; when a need exists, a tension is created that the dynamism then seeks to satisfy. The second category is made up of *interpersonal dynamisms,* which include behaviors related to the *self-system* (i.e., one's own sense of personality organization) and to groups of others (i.e., one's behavior toward other persons). The self-system is a dynamism that basically organizes and patterns our behaviors along certain lines; it defines certain behaviors as consistent with the way we see ourselves. By the same token, it excludes from awareness those experiences that are incongruous with our self-perceptions. Thus, to some degree the self-system can put blinders on us such that we do not see what we don't want to see. The self-system is formed by the messages we receive from others about how they see us, what Sullivan called *reflected appraisals.* Thus, "the mother who has labeled . . . her son as a 'wild animal' or 'bad boy,' to be broken and subdued, ensures by her continuing reflected appraisals of him that he will come to view himself in precisely these terms" (Rychlak, 1973, p. 257).

The interpersonal dynamisms also pattern the way we react to others and thus the way we think others see us. If we see others as perceiving us to be intelligent or charming, as opposed to incompetent or boorish, our behavior will be patterned accordingly. As with the zonal dynamisms, the interpersonal dynamisms serve to meet certain needs—specifically, interpersonal needs such as security, intimacy, and love. Indeed, all people pattern their experiences in certain ways, and thus we act and react according to certain expectations. This concept is not unlike Adler's proposal that we mold our lives according to certain ideas or lifestyles.

The second major concept introduced by Sullivan was that of *personifications*. These, too, are dynamisms, and they refer to one of our earliest developmental patternings of experience—namely, the images an individual has of him or herself or of another person. Thus, good boy, bad boy, good mother, bad mother, good adult, and bad adult are all images or ideas created during early development that serve to organize behavior. As you might guess, this concept is quite similar to Adler's idea of prototypes.

Sullivan called these personified images "eidetic people" because they create generalized classes of expectations from others who resembled the images in our memories. Thus, for example, the image of "good mother" may generate a positive attitude and resulting pattern of behavior in our relationship with older adult females. In essence, we act through these personifications in our interpersonal contacts.

Another type of personification is the tendency to assign human qualities to nonhuman, inanimate, or imaginary objects. Thus, our notion of pets as having certain personalities, or the concept of "Santa Claus," influences the patterning of our behavior under certain circumstances. The tendencies to pattern our interpersonal interactions according to eidetic people and to anthropomorphize are present in each of us, although they will be manifested differently in each case according to our personal, singular experiences.

A third basic concept introduced by Sullivan is the notion of *cognitive processes*. Sullivan believed that we process our experiences in different ways, depending on our psychological development and on the types of experience we have had. In developmental terms, the earliest and most primitive mode of cognitive processing is called the *prototaxic*; this refers to the experience of raw life and of physiological reactions, with little or no meaning for the experiencing person. Prototaxic experience is thus unconscious, occurring for the most part before the development of verbal abilities. However, prototaxic experience can continue to influence behavior throughout our lives, although to a lesser extent than in early childhood. A child, for example, might experience fear at the same time her mother expresses fear, almost as if the two were connected by an invisible umbilical cord. Likewise, an adult might experience a physiological reaction in the presence of another person, without understanding why.

As the child begins to learn to use language, he or she enters the *parataxic* mode of experiencing, a mode more advanced than the prototaxic in that it involves a basic ability to communicate with others. This cognitive process "consists of seeing causal relationships between events that occur at about the same time but that are not logically related" (Hall and Lindzey, 1970, p. 144). Thus, the parataxic mode is highly intuitive and may lead to interpretation of various signs in the environment as having special meanings for us but not for other people. Superstitious behavior is largely a parataxic way of thinking. Again, this type of experience affects us to some extent throughout our lives, as evidenced by our tendency, say, to assign a special meaning to a certain facial expression in another person or to subjectively interpret a particular event.

The last stage of cognitive processing, the fully matured stage, is the *syntaxic* mode of experiencing. At this stage, the use of language is mature and we use words that are consensually validated; that is, the meanings of the words we use are generally agreed upon by a number of people. Our ability to abstract continues to develop within this mode. It is this way of processing experience that characterizes most of our adult lives.

Defense Mechanisms

For Sullivan, anxiety referred to the experience of a threat to security. He designated the primary defense mechanism employed in dealing with anxiety as *selective inattention*, a process by which we may notice, but not pay attention to, objects or events that are not congruent with our self-system, that may cause it real or imagined harm, or that may hurt our self-esteem. In general, selective inattention becomes a problem only when our experiences become dissociated from the self—that is, when we deny or fail to acknowledge what we really do feel and sense. The latter condition is analogous to Freudian repression, in which experiences are withheld from conscious expression.

Sullivan recognized other defense mechanisms, but he saw them primarily as means of adjustment (Rychlak, 1973). He viewed Freudian sublimation, for example, as a substitution of socially accepted activity for a behavior pattern that yields anxiety and displacement as a deflection of one emotion from one context to another. And he viewed Adler's concept of compensation as a dynamism by which simpler activities are substituted for more difficult ones. Overall, for Sullivan, defense mechanisms represented alterations in patterns of behavior that have become ineffective or threatening.

Developmental Theory

Sullivan also proposed stages of development, many of which are analogous to the Freudian stages. However, in line with his concept of cognitive processes, Sullivan concentrated on the changes that take place in how we understand our surroundings and how these form the dynamisms that govern our behavior.

The first stage he called *infancy*, basically the period from birth to the maturation of language. Zonal dynamisms are active during this stage, and Sullivan saw them as filling primarily oral needs (as Freud would have proposed). Thinking is prototaxic in the early portions of this stage and gradually begins to evolve to the parataxic mode as language comes into increasing use.

The second stage is *childhood*, during which the use of language and the need for playmates mature. We also develop some sense of empathy at this time. Thus, during this stage, the syntaxic mode of thinking comes into being.

The third stage, the *juvenile* stage, spans the time from the need for playmates to the need for intimacy with others of our own sex. The self-system now begins to confront the world and to express a need for a close friend, a "chum," who can help us develop this dynamism. Competition with others also occurs at this time, a need occasionally in conflict with the need to be liked by others.

The fourth stage, *pre-adolescence*, ranges from intimacy with others of the same sex to the sparking of sexual attraction. The "chum" is an equal now in a two-person relationship, and shared genital desires begin to develop. Loving begins to emerge as the equivalent of giving to others.

The fifth stage, *early adolescence*, encompasses the period from the beginnings of the dynamism of sexual behavior to a patterning of that behavior. This patterning is now transferred to the opposite sex, and distinctions between lust and love needs begin to form in the new two-person interaction.

The last stage, *adolescence and maturity*, encompasses the rapid expansion of the syntaxic mode, which has been slowly developing since the childhood stage; at this time, the need for intimacy with at least one other individual grows stronger.

Sullivan's developmental stages, while reminiscent of Freud's clearly reveal the *social* nature of our experiences and perceptions. The dynamisms of self and of others form through growing and changing cognitive processes and interpersonal encounters. Failures during these developmental stages reflect frustrated individual needs, both zonal and interpersonal, and may bring about the formation of dynamisms that are ineffective or destructive.

In a therapeutic context, Sullivan felt that the maturing child must receive treatment for any poorly socialized views that may have developed. Sullivan's ideas are particularly cogent in this regard when we consider that the child forms his or her dynamisms, or views of self and others, within certain family patterns of behavior; the child learns to survive (i.e., to fulfill certain needs) based on how others behave toward him or her. Unfortunately, a number of families behave in idiosyncratic ways. From my own therapeutic experiences, I can attest to the common difficulty many individuals have in adjusting to the fact that the rest of the world is not like their family; in such cases, the dynamisms they have developed at home may be inoperative when dealing with the world at large.

APPLICATIONS IN HEALTH AND ILLNESS

Adler and Sullivan championed both the notion of personal responsibility for our behaviors and the importance of other persons in defining and forming our personalities. Both believed that the early formation of a lifestyle or self-system occurs through reflected appraisal (i.e., how others see us) and that this lifestyle generates a coherent, organizing principle underlying our behavior. The unconscious, they felt, represents that which is not understood, but they did not see it as exerting an independent, irresistible influence at variance with our conscious motives. Both theorists emphasized the maturing of a need for social interaction, loving, and giving as individuals develop.

In order to understand the individual patient from this perspective, we need to ask the following questions: What is the patient's lifestyle? How was it formed? What is likely to influence it? Both Adler and Sullivan subscribed to the principle of fictional finalism—in other words, that we live according to our ideas or personifications of reality rather than on the basis of reality itself. Thus, it is important to determine the patient's view of reality.

Using the categories described by Weinman (1981), we might also ask these questions: Are the patient's symptoms perceived as congruent with his or her lifestyle or self-concept? For example, might the patient have a self-concept that identifies him as sickly, dependent, and/or needing care from others? If so, the assertion by the health care professional that the patient's symptoms are not serious or require little attention might result in considerable resentment. On the other hand, if we are dealing with the young man described in the first chapter, whose personal style is that of a leader and self-determined person, then attempts at creating an effective, caring medical situation may prove extremely frustrating. It might be better to permit such a person to participate in making decisions to emphasize the preservation of strength and independence that will result from good medical care.

The ways in which individuals respond to symptoms will also have much to do with their perceptions of self and others. For example, it is well known that in socioeconomically disadvantaged communities, either inner-city or rural, there is strong mistrust of professional health care systems. It is not hard to understand how such a "medical dynamism" could develop, given that personalized, effective attention to health needs is not part of the general experience of people in these settings.

Lifestyles, as already mentioned, are also quite likely to have an impact on symptom formation. For example, the development of a self-system with little personal responsibility may lead to behaviors, such as smoking, drinking, and poor sleep habits, that increase the risk of a variety of diseases. How an individual responds to illness likewise reflects his or her lifestyle: a given person may persist in noncompliance with regimens, may continue at-risk behaviors, or may simply refuse to believe the medical advice given. The response of the director to his heart surgery in the movie *All That Jazz* provides a good example of how lifestyle can interfere with the way one deals with illness.

The response to medical treatment, aside from the above implications, must be considered in interpersonal terms. The physician, nurse, and other health care professionals may indeed trigger past associations in the patient, thus taking on the roles of father figure, loving mother, stern teacher, or other "eidetic people" in the patient's eyes. The patient's behavior in response may consequently have little basis in reality. The surprised professional, upon recommending treatment, may then find that the patient becomes angry for no apparent reason. It could be, in this case, that the patient sees a resemblance between the health care professional—an authority figure—and a parent with whom past interactions have been unpleasant and threatening.

Let me conclude this section by describing a patient from the standpoint of interpersonal personality theory. The patient was a young man with a two-year history of complaints of fever, backache, and fatigue associated with diagnosed chronic prostatitis. Yet he was disabled at work to an extent well beyond that expected by the nature of his illness. The patient expressed anger over this illness and blamed it on a girl with whom he had had sexual contact, calling her a tramp. In the course of our conversation, however, it became apparent that he himself had had numerous sexual contacts and saw himself as quite a ladies' man. His lifestyle was apparently one of general irresponsibility, but it included a self-system of being attractive and valued by others for appearance and wit. Upon psychological evaluation, the patient revealed numerous bodily concerns that reflected a genuine fear associated with any bodily dysfunction, which would severely threaten his concept of self. The association of bodily dysfunction with genital areas accentuated this threat since the patient's self-image was tied so heavily to sexual activity. The patient's back problems, resulting in disability from work, thus provided a convenient focus of his concerns and served to selectively remove from his attention the threats to his self-esteem. At the conclusion of his evaluation, the patient was informed by medical personnel that there was evidence of psychological contribution to his symptoms, and counseling for resolution of his personal conflicts was recommended. The patient followed through on the recommendations and returned to work soon thereafter.

In sum, the approach taken by Adler and Sullivan is in some ways easier to grasp than that of the analytic theorists and can often be applied quite directly to the individual. However, the most important contribution of the interpersonal approach, I believe, is the concept of the health care professional as part of an interpersonal interaction with the patient such that the dynamisms of both determine the quality and outcome of the medical situation. For a broader treatment of interpersonal aspects of health care, see Counte and Christman (1981), another volume in this series.

4

LEARNING APPROACHES

Learning is the process by which various responses or behaviors become associated with particular stimuli or cues. This association takes place according to certain rules, and it is the systemic organization of these rules that constitutes learning theory.

Although learning theory was developed in the laboratory through the study of observable behaviors, primarily in animals, it was soon adopted as an alternate way of looking at human behavior from that of postulating forces, structure, and topography in personality. Adherents of this approach are called *behaviorists*. Although many great strides in understanding human behavior were made by means of this approach, it is no longer seen as entirely explanatory in the absence of "reference to conscious phenomena" (Bakal, 1979, p. 204), that is, without considering how we think about things. However, in the field of medicine, behaviorist approaches are commonly employed because of their reference to specific antecedents of physiological and behavioral response and because of their adherence to principles of experimental evidence in demonstrating changes in these types of response. Although there are a large number of contributors and theories in this area, a notable few have dominated the field. In this chapter, we will concentrate on the theories of Pavlov (1927), Hull (1952), Dollard and Miller (1950), Skinner (1938), and Bandura (1969). Again, this chapter will provide a general introduction to the theories in this particular area; for more comprehensive study, the reader is referred to core personality texts, learning texts (e.g., Hilgard, 1956), and the authors' original works.

37

PAVLOV: CLASSICAL CONDITIONING

Before we begin our discussion of specific theorists, we must define a few terms common to most of their formulations, some of which have already been mentioned. A *response* is an activity that can be connected with an antecedent event through learning. A *stimulus* is any event to which a response can be connected. *Learning* is the situation in which the stimulus and response become connected. A *cue* is any event that takes on stimulus properties.

Pavlov (1927) described a form of learning in which the resulting behavior is controlled by events that preceded it. Such behavior is called *respondent behavior*; a specific reaction is a *conditioned response*. Generally, such behaviors or responses are naturally occurring reactions to appropriate environmental events that, through the process called *classical conditioning*, become associated with novel environmental events. (I use the terms *behavior* and *response* interchangeably here, but perhaps I should be more precise. Behavior is one type of response; a physiological reaction would be another.)

All types of response, as defined, are amenable to conditioning. The basic paradigm of classical conditioning is as follows:

(a) Unconditioned Stimulus (UCS) →→→ Unconditioned Response (UCR)
(b) Conditioned Stimulus (CS) + UCS →→→ UCR
(c) CS →→→ Conditioned Response (CR)

First, a natural reaction (UCR) occurs in response to a natural stimulus (UCS). In the classic (no pun intended) example of "Pavlov's dog," the UCR was salivation and the UCS was the sight of meat. Next, an unrelated stimulus (CS) is paired with the UCS; the UCR continues to occur. For Pavlov's dog, the CS was the sound of a bell. Following a sufficient number of pairings, the sound of the bell alone produces salivation in the dog; this response is now conditioned and is thus called the CR. The animal has learned to produce a naturally occurring response to an unnaturally occurring stimulus; dogs do not normally salivate at the sound of bells. The association of the bell and salivation is a form of learning accomplished through the process of classical conditioning.

There are several principles associated with this relatively straightforward paradigm that, while adding to its complexity, also explain how certain human behaviors can be accounted for. The first is *stimulus generalization*, which refers to the fact that the more an event resembles the conditioned stimulus, the more likely the conditioned response will occur. According to Rychlak (1973), for example, "a dog conditioned to salivate to a bell of a certain level of cycles per second (e.g., 1000) would *also* salivate, though perhaps to a lesser degree, to values approximating this level (e.g., 500 to 1500)." By the same token, if you condition a dog to salivate to the sound of an alarm clock, it might also salivate to the sound of a doorbell. A second basic principle is *response generalization*. This term refers to the occurrence of more than a singular response to a given stimulus. For example, the dog might blink its eyes or lick its chops when it salivates.

By selectively pairing the CS and UCS to produce a specific or generalized CR, we can increase or decrease stimulus or response generalization. Decreasing the generalization, that is, teaching an organism to be very specific in what it responds to, or in how it responds, is called *stimulus discrimination* and *response discrimination*, respectively. Therefore, if the initial conditioning paradigm were presented in such a way that only a bell of a certain tone were paired with food, the salivating dog would eventually produce the CR only to the intoned bell. Similarly, if the bell and food were removed whenever the dog engaged in a response aside from salivating the CR would eventually become highly specific.

When a classically conditioned response is established, how does one go about "disassociating" it from a particular stimulus? The process of doing so is called *extinction*. Extinction involves repeated presentations of the CS over time, in the absence of the UCS; eventually the CR will cease to take place. If we continue to ring the bell without presenting food, the dog will eventually cease salivating in response to the bell. As you might expect, the more strongly established the relationship between the bell and food, the longer it will take to disassociate the response of salivation from the stimulus of the bell by means of extinction.

HULL: DRIVE REDUCTION

Clark Hull's complex theory of learning basically maintains that associations between stimuli and particular behaviors are strengthened (reinforced) when they reduce some drive or need. Thus, behaviors such as obeying the call of a dinner bell are associated with the reduction of the hunger drive.

Hull's theory (1952) is far too complex to present in entirety here, but I will try to cover some of its most important contributions to the understanding of learning. One of Hull's basic concepts, as already mentioned, is *reinforcement,* that is, the strengthening of behavior. This strengthening occurs when a drive reduction takes place. *Primary reinforcement* refers to a basic, immediate reduction of drive, such as in the dinner bell example given earlier. However, we can clearly see that this contingency would account for, at best, only a minimal portion of our behaviors.

Hull described *secondary reinforcement* as addressing more complex behaviors. Such secondary reinforcement strengthens behaviors associated with primary drive reduction. For example, money earned for working at a job is a form of secondary reinforcement because it is associated with buying food, which results in a reduction of the primary hunger drive. Operating through complex networks of behaviors, secondary reinforcement can strengthen great varieties of apparently unrelated actions by distant associations to primary drive reduction.

A related concept is the *anticipatory goal response.* In conjunction with certain learned behaviors, such as coming to the supper table, we also learn associated behaviors, such as washing our hands or sitting in a particular chair. These behaviors, in and of themselves, do not lead to drive reduction, but they become associated with the particular behavior of eating, which does have this result. Thus, complex chains of behaviors can be evolved that are tied to relatively simple, singular drive-reduction behaviors.

The last aspect of Hull's theory we will address here is related to the complex chains of behaviors that develop in the individual, known as the *habit-family hierarchy.* As I have already pointed out, we seldom learn any one specific behavior, rather, we develop complex chains of behaviors, with particular behaviors most likely to occur regularly under given circumstances. This group of behaviors is the hierarchy of which Hull speaks. The hierarchy predicts which response is most probable when a given stimulus occurs; if that response is not successful in providing drive reduction, then a behavior lower down on the hierarchy—that is, a less probable behavior—will occur. It follows that if we hear the dinner bell, wash our hands, sit in our chairs at the table, and find that nothing happens, we might then begin inquiring after the food; if that fails to bring about the desired result, we might get up and go looking for it, and so on.

As mentioned earlier, this brief sketch of Hull's theory does no justice to its complexity, probably the most complex approach to learning developed by any one theorist. Partially because of its complexity, it has not had a major impact on current approaches to the conceptualization of behavior, especially as they relate to health care. However, the idea of drive reduction as a major impetus for learning is not at all alien to analytic dynamic notions of impulse or force; indeed, it was Hull's theory that provided the framework for a major attempt at integrating behavioral theory with more traditional analytic theory.

DOLLARD AND MILLER: AN ATTEMPT AT INTEGRATION

Dollard and Miller (1950) subscribed to the behaviorist notion that we can make only those responses we have learned and that we make them by necessity when the stimulus conditions are appropriate. They argued that cues, or events that take on stimulus properties, exert a strong influence over our behaviors that goes beyond the simple notion of stimulus and response association. They also suggested that the behaviors themselves can become cues that elicit further behaviors; that is, they become *cue-producing responses*. In this instance, a cue produces a certain response that in turn becomes a cue for another response, and so on. Such cue-producing responses are of two kinds: *verbal* (as in "Bring me that piece of cake") and *nonverbal* (such as a look, a glance, or a feeling). These behaviors can create a long chain of seemingly unrelated responses, one behavior building on the next. Although similar to Hull's notion of behaviors becoming associated in relation to a particular goal, Dollard and Miller's concept has expanded the way in which behaviors relate to one another by suggesting that one behavior may lead directly to another behavior without necessarily being directly related to a given goal. Language (the use of verbal cues) is the main cue-producing response; it develops through the labeling of various feelings, behaviors, and experiences. Complexity in language is introduced by the use of logic, the process by which rules for the effective use of verbal cues become established.

The chain of stimuli and behaviors between an original stimulus and final behavior might look something like this:

Stimulus →→ Response A
    ↓
    Cue →→ Response B
       ↓
       Cue →→ Response C
          ↓
          Cue →→ Response D
             ↓
             Cue →→ Final Reponse

A Stimulus, such as seeing a dish of ice cream in the freezer, might lead to Response A, salivation, which in itself becomes a cue leading to Response B, a worry about weight, which becomes a cue leading to Response C, a turning away from the refrigerator, which becomes a cue leading to Response D, feeling bad, which becomes a cue leading to the Final Response of calling a friend on the telephone.

Dollard and Miller incorporated much of Hull's theory in their description of the rules for how such connections between behaviors take place. However, they added many of their own unique contributions to the principles of behavior, contributions that were derived from their own independent studies. They included earlier notions of stimulus and response generalization in addressing Hull's notions of secondary reinforcement and anticipatory goal response. They also addressed the notion of frustration as being equivalent to a blocked drive. When frustration occurs, an innate anger response operates to remove the block to reinforcement, and thus drive reduction occurs.

Mowrer (1939) described how certain behaviors can be both anxiety-producing and self-reinforcing at the same time, when related to a particular drive. He translated this idea in terms of how we behave when faced with anxiety, after which Dollard and Miller incorporated this detail into their theory. Basically, Mowrer proposed that anxiety, a response, is attached to a previously neutral cue. For example, following an automobile accident, we may feel anxiety upon getting into the car. Behaviors that avoid the situation then take place, thereby reducing anxiety (a case of drive reduction; no pun intended), and these behaviors are thus reinforced, resulting in our refusal to drive a car.

With regard to efficiency in learning, Dollard and Miller proposed that immediate reinforcement is more effective than delayed reinforcement. This notion has led to a prediction in terms of certain behaviors: the more immediate the reinforcement, the more likely we are to elicit a particular behavior. Dollard and Miller called this phenomenon the *approach gradient*: the closer we are to a particular desirable goal, the more motivated we are to achieve it (the greater the drive). Thus, those behaviors associated with the drive reduction become more frequent. On the other hand, the closer we come to an aversive event, the more motivated we are (the greater the drive) to avoid it! This phenomenon is termed the *avoidance gradient*. Again, it follows that those behaviors associated with avoiding an aversive event become more frequent the closer we are to the event.

Employing the concepts of approach and avoidance gradients, Dollard and Miller discussed the conflicts we face in our daily lives that can be described in those terms. First is the *approach-approach conflict*; this is the situation in which we are attracted to two mutually exclusive events, such as going to a party and getting a good night's rest when we are very tired. (See Figure 4.) The two approach gradients pull equally at us and we tend to vacillate between one goal and another. However, the theory of approach gradients also suggests that if we begin to move toward one of the two events, the pull toward that event will become stronger and dominate the motivation toward the other event. Thus, if we are sitting at home plagued by indecision over whether to attend a party or stay at home, and we lie down in bed and begin a comfortable nap, it is more likely that we will stay at home altogether.

By the same token, we can become engaged in an *avoidance-avoidance conflict*, in which we must choose between one of two equally aversive events such as writing a research paper or studying for an exam (provided both are aversive to us). Again, in terms of gradients, the two push us away equally and we tend to be stuck in the middle, vacillating between both. However, unlike the previously described conflict, if we begin to move toward one of the two events, it becomes increasingly aversive and the other event becomes less

FIGURE 4. Difference between approach and avoidance choices. This is a schematic diagram of the gradients to approach (or to avoid) two stimulus objects, X and Y. If the two objects elicit only approach, the individual starting at P will be expected to go directly to X; if they elicit only avoidance, he will be expected to go away from X until he passes the point at which the gradients cross and then to turn back. It is only for the sake of simplicity that the gradients are represented by straight lines in this diagram. Similar deductions could be made on the basis of any curves that have a continuous negative slope. (From Dollard and Miller, 1950, Figure 18, p. 364. Reprinted by permission of McGraw-Hill Book Company and the authors.)

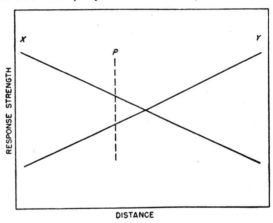

so; then we tend to move back toward the other event. Thus, when studying for the exam, working on the paper becomes the more attractive option (see Figure 4). In this way, we set up a vacillating pattern of behavior that is difficult to break out of.

A simpler but equally frustrating situation is the *approach-avoidance conflict*, which refers to our being equally attracted to and pulled away from an event—for example, being asked to work an overtime shift when we are tired and have other plans but still need the extra money. The gradients of approach and avoidance apply to one event, as can be seen in Figure 5, but as we come closer to the event, the avoidance gradient rises more steeply than does the approach gradient. Thus, although we may be initially attracted to an event, the event becomes more aversive as it nears, and we tend to become stuck again. In other words, as the overtime shift gets closer,

FIGURE 5. Simple graphic representation of an approach-avoidance conflict. The tendency to approach is the stronger of the two tendencies far from the goal, while the tendency to avoid is the stronger of the two near to the goal. Therefore, when far from the goal, the subject should tend to approach part way and then stop; when near to it, he should tend to retreat part way and then stop. In short, he should tend to remain in the region where the two gradients intersect.

It is only for the sake of simplicity that the gradients are represented by straight lines in this diagram. Similar deductions could be made on the basis of any curves that have a continuous negative slope that is steeper for avoidance than for approach at each point above the abscissa. (From Dollard and Miller, 1950, Figure 15, p. 356. Reprinted by permission of McGraw-Hill Book Company and the authors.)

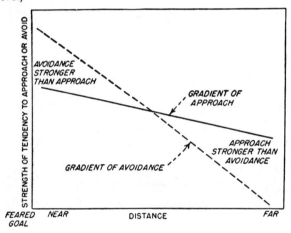

the more we wish we were doing something else – to the point where we try to get out of it.

The final conflict I will discuss here is among the most difficult to handle, the *double approach-avoidance conflict*. This conflict basically includes the aspects of both the approach-approach and approach-avoidance conflicts: We are simultaneously attracted to and pushed away from two mutually exclusive events. The rules for the approach-avoidance conflict apply to each event; therefore, the closer we get to one, the more its aversive aspects begin to dominate and the more attractive the other event becomes. Such a conflict may occur in the case of a diabetic individual who must manage her diet

45

strictly. If she does correctly manage her diet, her health is maintained; yet she also experiences the aversive aspects of not being able
to eat foods she wants. By the same token, she may eat the foods she
wants but will then experience the aversive aspects of deteriorating
health. Figure 5, if applied to two opposing events such as the more
simple approach-approach or avoidance-avoidance conflicts (Figure
4), graphically illustrates this conflict. As with the other conflicts, the
individual in double approach-avoidance conflict tends to vacillate
between approaching one event and avoiding the other and then
reversing the approach and avoidance. Treatment of patients caught
in this bind, such as the one with diabetes described above, can be
especially difficult for the health care professional.

Dollard and Miller used the principles of learning theory to
reinterpret analytic theory. In place of the pleasure principle as a
prime motivation for behavior, they substituted the principle of reinforcement, which holds that behaviors become associated with
stimuli because of their drive-reduction consequences. The unconscious, on the other hand, translates into those behaviors carried
into action without any labeling to identify them. Thus, according to
Dollard and Miller, non-verbal cue-producing responses may be
responsible for inefficient behaviors; one way to help the patient gain
control of these responses is to aid him or her in providing verbal
labels for them.

For Dollard and Miller, the conscious translates into those cue-
producing responses that have been learned throughout life and that
continue to function adequately—a concept also close in meaning to
that of the ego. The superego represents the complex rules of proper
behavior learned from parents, school, and other cultural contexts.
For example, a cue-producing response such as the idea that stealing
is "bad" may lead to the avoidance of theft behaviors.

Repression, the primary defense mechanism in analytic theory, is
seen as an automatic tendency to stop thinking and avoid remembering. In the context of learning theory, it represents an inhibition of
various cue-producing responses. Dollard and Miller identified three
types of repression. The first is the inhibition of those responses that
label a drive; non-verbal cue-producing responses influence
behavior particularly when the verbal labeling of those responses
would otherwise cause discomfort. For example, a woman's behavior
toward a certain man might be governed by an unpleasant reaction

46

to him based on his stimulus similarity to the woman's father; however, the labeling of this unpleasant reaction might be threatening to her image of her father, and thus the response remains unlabeled.

The second type of repression is the inhibition of responses that produce a drive; we tend to avoid those kinds of responses that we believe will result in undesirable behaviors. An individual may, for example, refuse to acknowledge anger for fear of negative consequences. The third type of repression is the inhibition of responses that mediate a drive. When we experience a reaction of anger, for example, certain other responses may also occur, such as an attempt to understand the situation; these latter responses in turn may lead to other kinds of behaviors, such as an attempt at discussion. Depending on the circumstances, then, certain kinds of repression can actually prove beneficial in our day-to-day lives.

Abnormal behavior was seen by Dollard and Miller (1950, pp. 222–226) as developing along the same principles as other kinds of behaviors, forming what is described as a *stupidity-misery cycle*. Basically, cue-producing responses are designated as "stupid" because they are unlabeled, or non-verbal. They often proceed from strong, unlabeled, emotional conflicts, which are usually of the approach-avoidance type. The resulting behaviors serve to reduce the conflicts, but they do not eliminate them; the obvious symptoms are thus self-defeating, and the individual remains miserable.

Dollard and Miller emphasized developmental processes in their theory to a greater extent than do other behavioral theorists, most of whom basically see development as the formation of increasingly complex relationships between stimulus and response. Dollard and Miller described four critical training situations during development that "can produce long-lasting effects on the character and habits of the individual" (1950, p. 132). The first is the *feeding situation*. This primarily involves the newborn infant, who is learning non-verbal cue-producing responses because he or she does not yet possess language. The reduction of hunger drives, social behaviors associated with feeding, and meeting of hunger drives through alternate means after weaning are all apsects of the important learning that takes place during this time.

The second situation is that of *cleanliness training*, which occurs during what Freud called the anal stage and is associated primarily with toilet training. In this case, also, learning takes place in the absence of fully developed language skills. Cleanliness training may be unpleasant for the child, particularly when it involves authority figures (parents) who enforce certain behaviors that are not specifically associated with any primary drive. Dollard and Miller implied (1950, p. 140) that waiting until the child has more capacity to develop verbal cue-producing responses might be an advantage in smoothing out toilet training.

Early sex training is the third critical developmental situation, related to masturbation (usually in the first year of life), sex-typing of personality (which is culture-dependent), attitudes about homosexual and heterosexual behaviors, and labeling of specific sexual conflicts. Failure to properly label responses, taboos on sex-related behaviors that are not sexually motivated (such as masturbation at the age of one year), and so on can lead to long-standing behavior problems involving stimuli related to sex.

Anger-anxiety conflicts characterize the fourth critical training situation, involving primarily the socialization of the response to frustration. Rivalry between young siblings is an example of a situation that provides a way of learning effective anger control in social situations; at a later age, anger may be modulated in response to parental acceptanc or rejection of certain anger-associated behaviors. It is also through verbally mediated cues that individuals learn to attach fears to certain cues that cause anxiety; these fears are typically related to feelings of anger, especially when anger is vigorously suppressed by the parents. Thus, if a child was severely reprimanded by her parents for hitting someone with a baseball bat, she might become afraid of playing baseball later on.

Overall, Dollard and Miller provided one of the most comprehensive frameworks for behavioral applications to personality theory. However, as with Hullian theory, Dollard and Miller's elegant approach has failed to be developed effectively since its introduction – most likely because of its complexity. Nevertheless, aspects of their theory continue to be invoked in the literature pertaining to human behavior.

SKINNER: OPERANT CONDITIONING

Probably the most popular and widely used behavioral approach is that of Skinner, the theory of *operant* or *instrumental conditioning.*

Skinner believed that a behavior, or response, is determined by the consequence that follows it. The basic principles and terms associated with operant conditioning can be understood without much difficulty. The first principle is that of *reinforcement*, defined as any event that increases the probability of the immediately preceding response in the presence of a given stimulus. *Positive reinforcement* occurs when the presence of an event increases the probability of the response, whereas *negative reinforcement* occurs when the absence of an event increases the probability of the response. Giving candy to a child for doing something is an example of positive reinforcement; not hitting a child for doing something is negative reinforcement. Both events have the same effect: they increase the probability of the immediately preceding behavior. *Punishment* occurs when the presence of an event *decreases* the probability of the immediately preceding behavior. Spanking a child who has misbehaved is an example of punishment.

From these basic principles, Skinner derived a complex theory of behavior, several aspects of which will be described here. However, certain additional principles need to be examined first. As already noted, we must provide reinforcement in order to produce a behavior. The production of behavior is accomplished through the process of *shaping*—that is, reinforcing first those behaviors that approximate the desired result, then those behaviors that are more like the behavior we want to produce, and finally the behavior itself. Thus, if we wish to teach a dog to sit, we would reward the dog first for standing still, then for bending the legs a bit, and finally for the actual behavior of sitting. As we reinforce the more specific behaviors, we begin to withdraw the rewards for the more general behaviors preceding them; in this way, behavior is shaped.

If, on the other hand, we wish to eliminate a behavior, we can choose from several options. One, of course, is to punish; but the problem with this approach is that it leaves the way open for too many other behaviors to occur. It is better to extinguish the undesired behavior and to reinforce the desired behavior. Extinction, as used by the operant behaviorist, is similar to the method employed by the classical behaviorist: in both cases, reinforcement for a particular behavior is simply withdrawn. If food is no longer given when a dog begs at the table, the dog will eventually cease to beg.

A common example of the practical application of these principles can be found in the situation of the misbehaving child. For many children, attention is a reinforcement for behavior. Thus, the child who throws a temper tantrum may actually have that behavior strengthened by the parent who yells at him, spanks him, or otherwise pays attention to the behavior. A far more effective means for dealing with temper tantrums is the procedure called *time-out* from reinforcement. In this procedure, a child throwing a temper tantrum is placed in an isolated room, away from all others, until the tantrum behaviors have ceased for a specified period of time (usually five minutes). Since it is impossible for the child to receive attention in this setting, the parent cannot inadvertently strengthen the undesired behavior. The time-out procedure is, of course, an example of extinction. Incidentally, we must keep in mind that when a reinforcement is removed from a given behavior, one of the first results observed is a temporary increase in the occurrence of that behavior. Since the behavior has been successful in obtaining a certain reward in the past, the first "logical" response to withdrawal of the reward is to intensify the behavior. Only after the behavior has failed for an extended period of time does the individual realize that the behavior itself must be changed. For this reason, many parents are discouraged in their use of time-out procedures: often, the first effect they notice is an immediate increase in the intensity and strength of the tantrum response. In fact, the first time-out they attempt may result in a tantrum lasting several hours. If applied consistently over time, however, this procedure will effectively extinguish the tantrum behavior.

Skinner also observed that the actual method of rewards presentation can have a significant impact on the strength of the behavior produced. The various methods available are categorized as *schedules of reinforcement* (Ferster and Skinner, 1957), in which both frequency and time can be varied. Frequency refers to the number of responses that occur before a reward is produced—after every response, after every fifth response, or after every tenth response, for instance. If the frequency is fixed, the schedule of reinforcement is defined as *fixed-ratio*; in this case, a predictable number of responses will produce a reinforcement. The schedule of reinforcement in which the frequency of response remains unpredictable is defined as *variable-ratio*; here, the individual knows a reward will occur following a number of responses but cannot determine exactly how many it will take.

An example of fixed-ratio reinforcement is the payment received for piecework, such as five dollars for every three newspaper subscriptions sold. Fixed-ratio reinforcement maintains steady behavior over time. Variable-ratio reinforcement, on the other hand, is exemplified by the casino slot machine: the player gambles on the chance that the "next" quarter will hit the jackpot but can never really be sure. As you may already realize, variable-ratio reinforcement schedules are extremely powerful in maintaining behaviors. The rates of behavior produced are generally higher and more difficult to extinguish than the rates produced under fixed-ratio reinforcement. This is because the individual has no way of predicting when a reinforcement will take place and thus has less information about when his or her behavior is no longer effective. The individual may ask him or herself "Will the next response produce a reward?"

The other varying factor in reinforcement schedules is that of time. In other words, a reward might be provided after a given period of time has elapsed, rather than on the basis of response frequency. A response that produces a reward every five minutes is operating under a *fixed-interval* reinforcement schedule. If on the other hand the response is rewarded after an unpredictable amount of time, the schedule of reinforcement is defined as *variable-interval*.

An example of fixed-interval reinforcement is a salary received regularly, such as every two weeks. A characteristic of this schedule is that the reinforced behavior tends to increase around the time the reinforcement is given, drops quickly towards zero level immediately following the reinforcement, and gradually increases again in the time before the next reinforcement is given. Indeed, we have all witnessed the phenomenon of busy activity as pay day approaches, followed by an immediate slowdown the day after. An example of variable-interval reinforcement, on the other hand, is the occasional bonus at work. We never know when it might be awarded, but we had bettter be producing at the time the recipients are chosen! This schedule, too, is quite powerful in maintaining behavior, although not as powerful as variable-ratio reinforcement. The variable-interval schedule also results in some dropoff of behavior immediately following the reward, but not to the same degree as seen in the fixed-interval schedule. See Figure 6 for a graphic representation of how schedules of reinforcement affect responses.

Operant conditioning techniques are generally straightforward in their application, and they produce effects on behavior that can be

FIGURE 6. Fixed-ratio, fixed-interval, variable-interval, and variable-ratio cumulative records. Characteristic cumulative response records for four partial schedules of reinforcement are shown here, based on trials of pigeons pecking at keys. Note two things about these records: First, the horizontal or vertical slashes on the response curves show when reinforcements were given. Second, although the record for each schedule is in several sections, the response curves are really continuous; the long response records have been cut and displaced on the chart to save space.

(a) The development of characteristic responding on a *fixed-ratio* schedule of partial reinforcement is shown here. The rate of response increases to a steady rate of about 3 responses per second. (b) The development of characteristic responding on a *fixed-interval* schedule of reinforcement is depicted in this record. Note the "scallops" in the final portion of the record. (c) The development of characteristic responding on a *variable-interval* schedule of reinforcement is shown here. Note that the reinforcement marks come at variable intervals. Note also the high, steady rate of response — especially in the 5th and 8th segments. (d) The high, steady rate of responding characteristic of *variable-ratio* schedules of reinforcement are displayed in this record. (From Morgan and King, 1971, Figure 3.13, p. 83. Reprinted by permission of McGraw-Hill Book Company and the authors.)

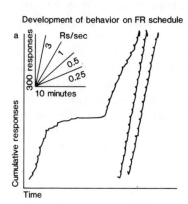

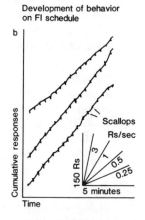

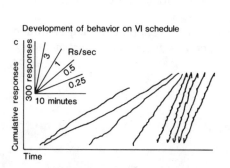

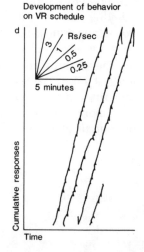

readily observed and measured. A currently popular application of these techniques in the field of health care is called *biofeedback*, which will be discussed briefly in the last section of this chapter. From the examples given, I am sure you can think of several other applications of these techniques in a variety of situations. Indeed, operant conditioning is the most commonly used behavioral approach in current psychological as well as medical treatments.

BANDURA: MODELING

The reader may have begun to wonder by now whether or not the behavioral approaches described in the previous sections can explain the immensely complex behaviors we witness every day. Regardless of the learning approach we are using, it seems a huge quantity of associational links between stimuli and responses would be required to account for the variety of behaviors we all possess. Bandura described what might be called a "better way" of describing learned behavior—*modeling*. This concept is known by other names as well, such as vicarious learning, observational learning, and imitation. Bandura (1969, p. 118) explained as follows:

> Virtually all learning phenomena resulting from direct experiences can occur on a vicarious basis through observation of other persons' behavior and its consequences for them. Thus, one can acquire intricate response patterns merely by observing the performances of appropriate models; emotional responses can be conditioned observationally by witnessing the affective reactions of others undergoing painful or pleasurable experiences; fearful and avoidant behavior can be extinguished vicariously through observation of modeled approach behavior toward feared objects without any adverse consequences accruing to the performer; inhibitions can be induced by witnessing the behavior of others punished; and finally, the expression of well-learned responses can be enhanced and socially regulated through the actions of influential models.

The concept of modeling is indeed a reasonable mechanism for understanding the learning of complex behaviors, without recourse to identification of every reinforcement, every mediating response, and so on associated with each stimulus we encounter. We *can* learn by imitating. A medical student, for instance, can more effectively learn to administer an injection by watching an expert do it correctly than by means of a shaping procedure (an approach I am sure the patient would highly object to). Modeling also provides an explanation of the acquisition of inappropriate behaviors due not to our own experience but to that seen in others. Thus, a child may have a fear of lightning because one of her parents has such a fear.

Several conditions are believed to influence whether or not an observed behavior will be modeled: (1) Increasing similarity between the model and the observer increases the probability that the model's behavior will be imitated. (2) The more probable it is that the model will be rewarded for his or her behavior, the more likely that the behavior will be imitated. (3) Increasing affective value of the model for the observer leads to increasing likelihood of modeling. ("Affective value" refers to the emotional importance for the individual. Thus, parents, bosses, leaders, and siblings may have important value for the observer in terms of power, financial security, national pride, and so on. The greater their value, the more likely their behavior will be copied.) (4) The more utility the modeled behaviors have for the observer, the more likely they will be imitated. (Watching someone perform a trapeze act may not stimulate imitative behavior, but watching someone fix a car is likely to do so.) (5) The complexity of the behavior to be modeled cannot exceed the capability of the observer to copy it, if the behavior is to be imitated. (6) Behaviors that can be "subdivided" by the observer will be more readily copied. (That is, when a model undergoes a series of motions or responses, the observer must be able to distinguish the components of that behavior in order to copy it. For example, swinging a baseball bat is easier to imitate if we understand how to hold the bat, how to poise the wrists, how to move the shoulders, and so forth.)

The above are only some of the general rules for increasing the probability that behaviors will be imitated (Bandura, 1969). However, they give a flavor for the kind of parameters that need to be considered if modeling approaches are to be used in understanding, changing, or initiating certain behaviors.

APPLICATIONS IN HEALTH AND ILLNESS

As mentioned at the start of this chapter, behavioral approaches have probably had the most significant impact on medical care of any theories of behavior. Although it is not possible to include all applications of these approaches in this chapter, I will discuss some basic examples of the general principles underlying each learning theory already covered. A more thorough discussion of these and other theories as they apply to health care situations can be found in Gordon (1981).

Classical Conditioning

As previously noted, classical conditioning (CC) usually involves a naturally occurring response that becomes associated with an unnatural stimulus. In the context of health care, this contingency frequently applies to autonomic nervous system responses, which are well-known to be susceptible to CC. For example, cardiac acceleration and blood pressure changes are common responses to a perceived threat (such as an automobile accident), and these responses can become associated with previously nonthreatening stimulus (such as getting into a car).

Let me give a specific example of how knowledge of the CC paradigm can be useful in the health care situation. A young patient of mine had developed a strong visceral reaction to the taste of Theophylline, a medication often used in treatment of asthma. The reaction was a strong one; the child vomited after ingesting the medication. After a few such instances, the child began to vomit at the mere sight of the medication bottle. The medical implications were significant: without the medication, the child would have to be hospitalized and possibly given medication intravenously. For a two-year-old child, this would be quite traumatic.

Using the CC paradigm, we can describe the visceral sensation as the unconditioned stimulus (UCS) and vomiting as the unconditioned response (UCR). It should be noted that the visceral sensation had not always resulted in vomiting; the child had previously taken the medication on numerous occasions without incident. But as a result of the few instances of vomiting, the visceral sensation became a conditioned stimulus (CS) leading to the conditioned response (CR) of vomiting; after a certain point, vomiting occurred each time the sensation was experienced. Soon thereafter, the taste of the medication and even the sight of the bottle became associated with the visceral sensation through stimulus generalization.

As described in the section on CC, extinction is the most appropriate method for eliminating a conditioned response. Accordingly, the medicine was then given repeatedly to the child until the vomiting ceased, that is, until there was nothing left to vomit. After several such episodes, the vomiting ceased and the child was able to take the medication successfully, thereby returning to the original and more healthy pattern of behavior.

A more common example of CC involving children, and a problematical one for health care personnel, is the acquired fear of doctors and nurses. Children often associate a visit to a medical office with pain previously experienced during injections, treatment for burns, and so on. Eventually, a white uniform or the appearance of a medical device can become a conditioned stimulus for the fear response. This association is especially pronounced if the child has been seen at the health facility only under painful circumstances; such a child would have good reason to be afraid.

In an attempt to diminish this problem, many pediatricians have arranged their offices and waiting rooms in such a way as to be less easily generalizable to a painful situation; that is, with the simple addition of small furniture and toys, they have effectively minimized stimulus generalization. Additionally, many health care professionals who deal with children dress less traditionally, having discovered that white uniforms are often associated with discomfort and fear. Overall, the best method of changing the conditioned response of fear in health care situations is that of extinction. The child who visits a health facility for regular checkups or for minor illnesses will gradually learn that pain is not always associated with the visit. In this way, the link between the conditioned stimulus and the fear response is weakened.

We have seen how easily an association can be established through classical conditioning to a number of naturally occurring reactions, often with serious medical implications. An understanding of the parameters influencing such behavior is therefore of great value in the health care situation.

Drive Reduction

As stated earlier, one factor determining the occurrence of a particular behavior in the presence of a given stimulus is the effectiveness of that behavior in reducing a drive. This connection can be applied to numerous situations in health care; let us consider just one.

A patient develops a pattern of taking analgesics when he experiences pain. Although this pattern may have originated during a period of severe pain, it is now a serious habit, occurring when the patient feels any pain—even minor aches. The stimulus is pain, the drive is to reduce pain, and the behavior satisfies the drive. The stimulus of severe pain has become generalized to include minor aches, and a habit-family hierarchy has been established in which the preferred response is to take analgesics. Such a situation is commonly encountered by health care personnel.

One possible solution to this problem of drug overuse is to change the habit hierarchy by reducing the drive through alternate means. In this connection, exercise (often prescribed for patients with low back pain) or relaxation (recommended for those with headaches) may provide an alternate way of reducing pain without adverse consequences; meanwhile, a new habit hierarchy can be established. A similar approach is employed in the current practice of patient instruction, in which patients are taught coping responses to stress (see Bieliauskas, 1982). In both cases, patients are learning effective ways of reducing the drive to avoid pain. In addition, patients can be taught to discriminate different levels of pain (stimulus discrimination), so that they are better able to identify what experiences initiated the drive. This is achieved by designating various scales or points of reference for the pain. For example, patients might be taught to view their current pain as a continuum, comparing it, say, to the pain of a pricked finger, of a bee sting, and of a burn. These perceptions will be different for each person and thus need to be dealt with individually. Ultimately, the patient will have learned to discriminate the experience that prompts drive reduction behaviors from an experience that is minor.

Such an approach may appear to be simple. Like the CC paradigm described earlier, however, it is actually quite complex and requires close attention to many parameters of behavior. Nevertheless, the principles of drive reduction theory can be very useful as guidelines in determining the influences on and effective interventions for problematic health-related behaviors.

The Dollard and Miller Integration

The examples already given for drive-reduction theory could, of course, apply to Dollard and Miller's integration of behavioral and analytic approaches as well. Let us now look at an illustration of one further portion of their theory, the concept of labeling as a cue-producing response and its applications to the health care setting.

Schacter and Singer (1962) proposed that when individuals experience physiological arousal for which there is no immediate explanation, they will label it and describe their feelings according to that label. A given feeling might be described as either joy or jealousy, depending on how it is labeled. If on the other hand the individual knows the appropriate explanation for the arousal, then further evaluations are not necessary. Schacter and Singer tested their propositions in a group of subjects, all of whom received adrenaline but were told that they had taken vitamins. Some subjects were told what to expect in the way of physiological reactions; others were not. Those subjects who were not so informed readily attributed a variety of emotional labels to their experience, whereas those who had been informed exhibited little need to evaluate their experiences. I have witnessed non-experimental cases of adrenaline administration (such as for an allergic response) in which the patients were not informed of the action of the catecholamine and became fearful and worried, not understanding what was being experienced. Fear is thus a labeled emotion, leading to further anxiety, pacing, and so on. This example points up one important aspect of all medical procedures: the necessity of explaining to the patient what is being done and what will be experienced. Without such an explanation, the patient is likely to mislabel a procedure or a reaction and may consequently develop behaviors that are harmful to the health care situation. A patient from whom blood is drawn, for instance, will react quite differently if she has been told that certain assays are being run than if she believes a medical student is drawing her blood for practice.

Operant Conditioning

The theory of reinforcement has been applied in two basic ways to health care. The first involves the study of how undesirable or desirable behaviors become established in patients or potential patients. On the one hand, Mikulic (1971) found that nurses in a particular setting inadvertently reinforced dependent behaviors in their patients; that is, they strengthened their patients' tendency to demand that everything be done for them. On the other hand, Gentry (1977) described a variety of studies that examine reinforcement techniques for increasing compliance with medical regimens. Reinforcement approaches have also been successfully employed in altering the behavior of patients with back pain (Fordyce, 1976; Sternbach, 1974) and even those with neurological disease (Montgomery and Cleeland, 1980). Punishment, too, has been demonstrated as a successful means of terminating certain destructive behaviors, such as life-threatening vomiting in children (Lang and Melamed, 1969).

The other area of impact involves the management, through operant conditioning, of various physiological responses of the body. The most popular method of physiological management is *biofeedback*, defined as "the use of electronic monitoring instruments to record and display physiological processes within the body" (Bakal, 1979, p. 228). In short, these instruments provide the patient with information that was not available before. Thus, for example, muscle contractions leading to tension headache can be connected to a tone that increases in pitch with increasing tension and vice versa. The pitch of the tone then becomes a positive reinforcer for behaviors that serve to decrease muscle contraction and thus relieve the headache. At present, since most applications of biofeedback involve the teaching of relaxation responses, there is some question as to whether a genuine reinforcement effect is taking place or whether the patient is just generally learning to relax (Belar, 1978; Cohen, McArthur, and Rickles, 1980; Silver and Blanchard, 1978). Nevertheless, biofeedback methods have been successfully employed for a variety of patient symptoms, including headaches, high blood pressure, epileptiform EEG activity, and peripheral vascular temperature, and have proved effective even in neuromuscular retraining following stroke. See Williams and Gentry (1977) and Schwartz and Beatty (1977) for a more thorough presentation of the varieties of operant conditioning and other behavioral interventions in medical settings.

Modeling

The primary applications for modeling in health care have involved the instruction of patients in certain kinds of behavior. For example, Melamed and Siegel (1975) were able to reduce hospital and surgical anxiety in children by means of a film demonstrating medical procedures and successful coping responses in young patients.

Hospitals now routinely show such films in pediatric units, as well as in adult units when procedures such as wound care, aspects of hygiene, and compliance with medical regimen must be taught. Basically, the patients learn, by imitation, how to be *effective* patients. The effectiveness of the models in such films in producing certain behaviors will be related to the principles outlined in the section on modeling.

Overall Individual Considerations

Learning theory approaches lend themselves quite directly to the analysis suggested by Weinman (1981), which was described in the first chapter. Symptom perception can be directly related to labeling processes. Symptom action can be understood in terms of either drive reduction, operant conditioning, or modeling approaches. Symptom formation can take place according to a number of rules, which can be viewed differently according to different learning theories. Similarly responses to illness and treatment can be related to the principles of learning theory.

Often, the same behavior can be understood in a number of different ways, according to different approaches. Of greater importance is that the approach taken leads to the most effective way of dealing with any given patient. Overall, the various learning theories have relatively straightforward applications to health care problems and thus have attained current popularity in applied medical settings.

COGNITIVE APPROACHES

The last theoretical approaches to understanding personality we will discuss are those of the cognitive theorists. The cognitive perspective concentrates on the individual's view of the world as the main determinant of his or her behavior. The cognitive theorists thus rely heavily on the notion of fictional sources for behavior—that is, on the individual's perceptions of reality—in their efforts to understand behavior.

Cognitive theories developed as a reaction against the beliefs that complex human behavior could be adequately described in terms of stimulus and response, unconscious motivation, or purely social influences. In a review of behavioral therapies, for example, Murray and Jacobsen (1971) emphasized the importance of such cognitive factors as awareness and conscious information processing in determining human responses to various learning tasks. In this connection, Spence (1966) reported that, in a classical conditioning study involving the eyeblink as a conditioned response, the subjects eventually realized "that their eyeblink had been conditioned, and immediately adopted a set not to blink to the conditioned stimulus" (Murray and Jacobsen, 1971, p. 711). Thus, a researcher's prediction of a particular response can be either short-circuited or enhanced by the subject's awareness of the behavioral contingencies present. It is, in part, this factor of awareness to which Dollard and Miller previously referred in the context of consciousness—that is, awareness of the verbal labeling of particular responses and the use of this labeling to guide further behavior (see Chapter 4).

Among the best developed cognitive theories of personality are those provided by George Kelly (1955a, 1955b) and Julian Rotter (Rotter, 1954; Rotter, Chance, and Phares, 1972). Through construct

61

theory, Kelly attempted to understand how our personal formulations about the world are formed and changed. By means of social
learning theory, Rotter attempted to blend cognitive and behavioral
theory in studying the formulation of personality through our interactions with others. Only a cursory introduction to these theories can
be provided here. The reader is referred to basic texts in personality
or to the authors' original works for a more thorough explanation of
their work.

KELLY: CONSTRUCT THEORY

A *construct*, according to Kelly, is "an identifiable, patterned
structure or style of viewing life" (Rychlak, 1973, p. 475) – in other
words, the hypotheses we hold about why things are a certain way
and what we can expect when we do certain things. On the necessary assumption that these interpretations of reality are subject to
revision – an assumption Kelly termed *constructive alternativism* – we
must continually test them and alter those that prove incorrect.
Therefore, we live in a world in which we can adjust and change,
rather than in a world of frozen, rigid givens. By the same token, according to Kelly, every individual can be considered a scientist who is
continually performing experiments on his or her conceptions of
reality.

As conceptual structures imposed on subsequent events, constructs are much like controls. There is a tendency in all of us to order
life around several controlling constructs, as well as a continual effort
to systematize our own personal constructs by minimizing the con-
tradictions between them. Constructs are thus ordinal in nature; that
is, some are more important than others. A *superordinate construct*,
(e.g., "I am a religious person") subsumes a *subordinate construct*
(e.g., "I will not steal"). In general, it is more difficult for us to alter
superordinate constructs than subordinate ones.

Constructs can also be described as loose or rigid, and we can
tighten or loosen them depending on the circumstances. Permeable
constructs are those that can take new elements into their organization. Overall, the concept of constructs pertains to how easy or how
difficult it is for us to change the way we look at the world and how
effectively we can adjust to new elements in our surroundings.

Kelly viewed the *self* as a core construct that exerts control over what we do and experience. The self is thus a superordinate construct that governs the formation and operation of subordinate constructs. Kelly also saw the self as a *role* construct. He defined role formation as a process in which the individual construes the construct processes of others, reaches an understanding of how they relate to him or herself, and thus becomes able to engage in interpersonal activity. The roles of nurse and patient are examples of such role constructs. The self is also seen as a *core role* construct in that it defines one's interpersonal interactions to a greater extent than do occupation constructs.

Kelly further described constructs as bipolar in nature. As you may recall, Jung, who advanced the theory of opposites in the formation of human personality, proposed that all conscious entities with which we identify also have their opposites, which we disavow. Kelly likewise saw bipolarity as an inherent characteristic of constructs, such that when we categorize experiences in a particular way, we also deny alternative constructs. It is this bipolar nature of the self construct that contributes to our understanding of how we are like or different from others.

When a construct is about to change—that is, when it begins to lose its structure—we experience *anxiety*. Anxiety occurs throughout our lives as our views of the world undergo continual alteration; it is the uneasy feeling we have when our previous, and familiar, ways of seeing things are challenged. The feeling of anxiety continues until a new construct is established to accommodate our new experiences. Ultimately, each of our personalities is formed according to the constructs formulated throughout our lives. Social factors influence these formulations along the way to the extent that society and culture validate or invalidate our constructs. Abnormality, as defined by Kelly, occurs when certain constructs are used repeatedly despite consistent invalidation.

Personal change, according to Kelly's construct theory, is accomplished through alteration of invalid constructs. For instance, an individual might acquire, by means of more effective constructs, the ability to predict and anticipate events. This viewpoint goes considerably beyond stimulus-response theory. Thus, when dealing with individuals in psychotherapy, Kelly would primarily look for solutions i.e., effective constructs and/or attempt to discredit invalid ways of looking at things. Often, he would advise an individual to behave "as if" certain constructs about the world were true, thereby encouraging the individual to try out a new role and see if it were more satisfactory.

Construct theory is distinctly human in its orientation and thus appeals to those who view human behavior as too complex to be explained in terms of sexual impulses, basic drive fulfillment, or simple reinforcement. The concept of the construct lends itself readily to interpersonal approaches to understanding behavior; indeed, there is much about it that may remind us of Adler's fictional finalism or Sullivan's reflected appraisals. We might also make the case that our cognitive constructs are learned responses and that these guides to our behavior follow the basic rules of learning.

ROTTER: SOCIAL LEARNING THEORY

Social learning theory (SLT) maintains that "the unit of investigation for the study of personality is the interaction of the individual and his meaningful environment" (Rotter, Chance and Phares, 1972, p. 4). What is stressed by this theory is our understanding of the situation in which we find ourselves, on the basis of which we can make some predictions about behavior. More specifically, as its name implies, SLT concentrates on learned behavior in the context of interactions with the environment. From this viewpoint, our past experiences are believed to influence present experiences, and thus our individual personalities are seen to have a unity. Behavior is described as goal-directed (i.e., certain reinforcements can be expected based on experience), which leads to the supposition that it is not just what is actually occurring around us but what we expect to occur that governs our behavior. In short, cognitive factors are seen by social learning theory to play a significant role in generating behavior.

This theory, although quite complex, is based on four basic concepts. The first is *behavior potential*, which refers to the probability of any behavior occurring in any given situation as calculated in relation to any life situation. Behavioral potential is thus a relative concept, in that a particular behavior has a probability relative only to other behaviors available to the individual. This behavior potential includes both overt behaviors, those that can be seen and easily measured, and covert behaviors, those that cannot be directly observed.

The next basic concept, that of *expectancy*, concerns a given behavior potential—namely, the probability held by an individual that a particular reward will occur as the result of a specific behavior in a specific situation. Stressed here is the subjective expectation held by an individual that performing a particular action will result in a particular consequence. Past experience plays a heavy role in such expectations. The more novel a situation is, however, the less influence expectancy can have on behavior potential since the individual in a new situation does not know what he or she can expect.

Reinforcement value, another concept associated with behavior potential, refers to the degree of an individual's preference for a particular reward to occur when the possibilities of occurrence of all alternative rewards are equal. This is also a relative concept in that it is defined in relation to other rewards; if one has a quarter, is he more likely to buy a candy bar, to buy an ice cream cone, or to keep the quarter in his pocket? Reinforcements can be internal (such as the satisfaction of saving) or external (getting something good to eat). Reinforcement value also depends on the type of need, be it a physical need (such as hunger) or a psychological need (such as discharging tension). Whether a reinforcement is immediately available or will be delayed as a consequence of behavior is also a determining factor in reinforcement value. (In other words, is a bird in the hand really worth two in the bush?)

Rotter provided a basic formula for the relationship of behavior potential to expectancy and reinforcement value:

$$BP = f(E + RV)$$

where behavior potential (BP) is a function (f) of expectancy (E) plus reinforcement value (RV). The values described by this formula will vary, of course, depending on when it is applied. If we apply it to the example given earlier of the quarter, it will make a difference if the decision is to be made in the morning before an important meeting or on a hot, lazy afternoon. What governs the overall application of the formula is the fourth major SLT concept, the *psychological situation*. By this is meant the internal and/or external stimulation being experienced by the individual at a given time. Each psychological situation is composed of cues that serve to arouse certain expectations in the individual for certain reinforcement values. In a given psychological situation, then, the individual can predict behavior potential if he or she knows the expectancy and reinforcement values that apply to it.

As you can see, SLT is of tremendous heuristic value to personality theorists, in that it generates specific predictions that can be tested experimentally and thus provides a means for organizing some of our knowledge about behavior in a meaningful way. (A large body of this research is discussed in Rotter, Chance, and Phares (1972).)

Nevertheless, human behavior is so complex that even SLT cannot completely encompass either the variety of behavioral possibilities open to the individual or the variety of experiences and internal responses that influence the final measurable behavioral outcome. An attempt to create an appropriately complex formula to account for the many vagaries of human behavior would run into the same difficulties as those experienced by Hull and his colleagues, who attempted as much with drive reduction theory. In the final analysis, although SLT can effectively predict certain behaviors in restricted situations, it is not always so effective in the less structured clinical situation. Still, it does provide a good vehicle for organizing our thoughts about a given patient in a medical situation. By paying close attention to the patient's values in life, to the patient's fears, and to the patient's behavior capacities relative to his or her past behavior, we can predict, with some assurance, what that patient is likely to do in a given situation in the future.

APPLICATIONS IN HEALTH AND ILLNESS

To repeat, cognitive theories urge us to pay particular attention to the way in which a patient perceives what is going on around him or her, so as to best understand the behavior we observe in that patient. Perhaps one of the best examples of how such an approach applies in the medical situation is the series of studies by Janis (1958) on surgical patients. Janis found a relationship between the amount of preoperative fear exhibited by surgical patients and their postoperative adjustment; that is, patients with a low amount of fear adjusted most poorly, those with moderate levels of fear adjusted most successfully, and those with the highest levels of fear were intermediate between the first two groups in their degree of adjustment. Thus, the presence of occasional concern and tension over specific aspects of the operation appears to be a good preparatory situation for the patient, but constant cheeriness and denial of all concern, as well as constant concern over matters of pain, mutilation, death, and so on, are less conducive to good surgical outcome. Janis also found that information given to patients prior to surgery had a significant impact on their level of fear. Patients with a low level of fear, it turns out, had little or no idea of what to expect about the procedure they were to undergo. We can therefore conclude that it makes sense to give patients appropriate information prior to surgery, as a beneficial factor in their eventual recovery.

Egbert, Battit, Welch, and Bartlett (1964) performed a study to test precisely this notion. Patients admitted for abdominal surgery were given either standard information about their operation *or* detailed explanations of the type of pain they were to experience, assurances of normal consequences of the operation, and reassurances of support in addition to the standard information on the night before surgery. Throughout the 5 days following surgery, the latter patients needed only half the sedation required by the other group of patients, and the informed patients went home an average of 2.7 days earlier than the noninformed patients.

From the perspective of cognitive theory, we are helping the patient define certain constructs to explain events (à la Kelly) when we provide information that can be incorporated into the role of "being a patient." In this way, anticipated pain, sensory distortions, and so on become a part of the patient's construct, which in turn alleviates the anxiety that would otherwise occur if the patient's preconceived notions about surgical discomfort were *not* matched by the actual experience. By the same token, a patient's expectancies of what will be experienced *following* surgery (à la Rotter) are clearly shaped by the information given prior to the operation. Again, a prediction of the behavioral potential in a psychological situation of preparedness will be quite different from that given in a psychological situation of confusion or uncertainty. The reader may recall that novel situations are least affected by expectancy (as Rotter's paradigm suggests); thus, information given to a patient in advance decreases the novelty of the experience and increases the desired effects of expectancy.

Further discussed in another volume in this series (Bieliauskas, 1982) is the importance of information in the prediction and control of stressing situations. Surgery is an example of such a situation. In general, the health care professional is advised to "tell the patient what is in store for him, specifically, what sensory experiences he will undergo (what he will see, feel, or hear); what he may see when he awakens from the operation, especially if he is to spend time in the recovery room; and so forth" (Strain and Grossman, 1975, p. 132). Indeed, cognitive theories present the operative rationale for taking such action.

Of course, surgery is only one example of the problems encountered in dealing with a patient's anticipatory ideas about medical care. For many individuals, even a brief examination is a novel experience. Here, too, efforts at aiding individuals in understanding what will happen to them, what tests and procedures mean for them, and so on are sure to result in less disruptive or inefficient behavior on the part of the patient. An analogy can be drawn between these efforts and the use of modeling techniques discussed in the previous chapter: indeed, the notion of preparing patients to be patients parallels the technique associated with cognitive theory in which the patient is helped to create effective role constructs and/or expectancies. A further discussion of systemic approaches in this context can be found in Melamed and Siegel (1980).

In terms of Weinman's (1981) categories, cognitive approaches are readily applicable to the process of understanding how a patient perceives symptoms; that is, the construct in which those symptoms are placed will determine whether they are seen as serious or incidental. The individual's response to the symptoms will depend on what current psychological situation is impinging on the expectancies and on the values associated with the consequences of a given behavior.

Proneness to certain symptoms and syndromes is best addressed by cognitive theory in the context of a particular cognitive structure or expectancy associated with a high-risk lifestyle. Such a lifestyle might involve, for example, a role structure of masculinity, which, if associated with smoking and alcohol consumption, would likely lead to increased risk of a variety of illnesses. Cognitive understanding of behavior is highly relevant to an individual's response to illness, as has already been discussed in terms of information supplied to patients about their illnesses and the medical procedures to be used in their treatment. Similarly, the response to treatment will be influenced by the construct of "being a patient" and by the expectancy of the situation formed from past experience. Overall, cognitive theories provide a significant tool in dealing with certain patient characteristics—namely, their perceptions of what it means to be sick and their anticipations about what will happen to them once they come under the care of a professional.

INDEPENDENT CONCEPTS

Apart from the various integrated theoretical approaches, a number of relatively atheoretical concepts of personality have emerged that have particular relevance to medicine. These concepts do not require that we make assumptions about either the organization of behavior or the motives and causes of behavior. Rather, they are descriptions of particular characteristics of behavior that reflect, in an experimentally documented and reliable fashion, the ways in which patients react to and/or influence the course of their illnesses. In other words, each concept describes a particular dimension of behavior and the ways in which that dimension affects the symptoms presented to the health care professional.

AUGMENTERS AND REDUCERS

Petrie (1967), for example, described a dimension of personality based on sensory experience. This type of experience is the tendency in each of us to respond to sensation to a greater or lesser degree, that is, to feel something more or less intensely relative to the experience of another person. Individuals can be characterized along this dimension in three ways: (1) The *reducer* is an individual who tends to subjectively decrease what is perceived; (2) the *augmenter* is one who tends to increase what is perceived; and (3) the *moderate* is one who neither reduces nor augments what is perceived. Common sense tells us that objects appear bigger or smaller, brighter or duller, rougher or smoother depending on certain unknown characteristics that are not the same in each of us. We can measure these characteristics by using standard stimuli, such as a pair of calipers open to a certain angle or different sized wooden spheres, to compare how people perceive them (as wider or narrower, larger or smaller, and so on). After gathering a number of such measures, we can determine whether a given individual tends to be an augmenter, a reducer, or a moderate. A fuller description of such measures can be found in Petrie (1967).

Of particular interest to the field of health care is the documented fact that individuals who are characterized as reducers exhibit a greater tolerance for pain. Such individuals appear to minimize painful stimuli in addition to other types of stimuli. In an experimental situation in which heat is applied in ever-increasing amounts, for instance, individuals who are reducers tend to tolerate more heat.

An additional finding reported by Petrie (1967) is that individuals who are most tolerant of pain are also the least preoccupied with signs and symptoms of health as measured by personality tests (see Chapter 8). These individuals appear to be relatively less sensitive to minor aches and pains; they subjectively pay less attention to health-related matters. Of course, such lack of attention may not always be in the best interests of health, especially in the case of illnesses that present with subtle symptoms. For example, I know of certain physicians who, upon experiencing mild symptoms of a heart attack, immediately engaged in excercise (such as push-ups). These individuals were not unaware of the implications of such symptoms; they had been trained as health care professionals, after all. Rather, they interpreted the experience of mild chest pain as muscular stiffness resulting from insufficient mobility, instead of seeing it as a sign of illness. The purely subjective interpretation of pain is the crucial factor here, as distinct from the concept of pain threshold. In a study demonstrating this phenomenon (Klepac, McDonald, Hauge, and Dowling 1980), college students were asked to describe themselves as either highly fearful or nonfearful of dental and nondental pain. The two groups exhibited no differences when pain threshold was measured by tooth pulp stimulation and electrodermal stimulation. However, the high-fear group reported more subjective pain from tooth pulp stimulation than did the low-fear group.

Certain medical practices also appear to function as reduction agents. Alcohol, for example, is well known to reduce pain and can thus be used to increase pain tolerance. Aspirin likewise increases pain tolerance as does audio analgesia. In this last procedure, the patient is provided with a white noise stimulus, the theory being that such overstimulation will automatically cause the patient to "shut down" external stimulation in general, including the experience of pain. Audio analgesia has been used with particular success by dentists.

In addition to the use of various drugs and the process of audio analgesia, certain other behavioral interventions can be employed to alter the perceptions of pain. One of the most popular methods is that of hypnosis, in which relaxation and imagery (the picturing of various perceptions in nonstandard ways, such as imagining a pain as an itch) are used to diminish the perception of pain. Hypnotic techniques are also currently being used to alter perceptions of other unpleasant medical effects such as those produced by burn treatment procedures (Achterberg, Kenner, and Lawlis, 1982) and the nausea resulting from cancer chemotherapy (Redd, Andreasen, and Minagawa, 1982). The notion of an augmenting and reducing dimension thus holds significant promise for understanding and dealing with behaviors associated with pain and other distress in health care procedures.

INTERNAL-EXTERNAL LOCUS OF CONTROL

The dimension of internal versus external locus of control concerns the distinction between experience (rewards or punishments) perceived as somehow influenced by ourselves (i.e., at least partially under our own control) and experience perceived as the result of forces beyond our control. The notion of internal organization and motivation for our behavior goes back at least as far as Allport (1937, 1961, 1962), who asserted that various dispositions within each of us account for the consistency seen in our behaviors—a consistency that defines us as individual personalities. Basically, the dimension of locus of control defines whether or not an individual feels any personal responsibility for what happens in his or her life. This feeling, in turn, will lead to particular kinds of behaviors. The person with an external locus of control is likely to interpret a health problem as the result of "germs" or "poisons" and come to a health care professional with the request that it be "fixed." Furthermore, it will be difficult to convince such an individual that illness can be avoided or cured "salutogenically," that is, through abstinence from cigarettes and alcohol, and so on. On the other hand, the person with an internal locus of control may avoid the physician altogether when feeling ill because "the doctor can't do anything, anyway" or "If I wait long enough, it will get better by itself." Such a person takes personal responsibility for his or her experiences but may neglect important external help when it is necessary. Salutogenic behaviors, however, are more likely to be faithfully followed by this type of individual. Kobasa (1979), for example, found that groups of upper- and middle-level executives who were less frequently ill, but were under the same amount of stress as executives who were more frequently ill, had an internal locus of control associated with a strong commitment to self, a vigorous attitude toward the environment, and a sense of meaningfulness about life.

The determination of which locus of control an individual can be identified with is generally accomplished by means of a test designed for this purpose, the Internal-External Locus of Control Scale (Lefcourt, 1973; Rotter, Seeman, and Liverant, 1962). This test is a self-report scale (see the section on Objective Tests in Chapter 8) listing examples of internal and external control of events to which an individual responds as being true or false. A test item might take this form: "What happens to me is my own doing." After a number of such items are designated as true or false, they can be scored and summed to provide a measure of internal or external locus of control for the individual in question.

Aside from providing a general prediction of health-related behaviors and styles, the locus of control dimension can be used to predict the probability that a given medical intervention will succeed with a given patient. In the last chapter, we discussed the importance of providing information to the patient about illness and medical procedures. Research on the locus of control dimension suggests that such medical information can be employed by patients in a way that relates to their perception of control over events. In this connection, Cromwell, Butterfield, Brayfield, and Curry (1977) studied coronary care unit patients who were either given or not given the opportunity to participate in the treatment and monitoring of their own conditions. They were also measured for locus of control. During the study, 6 of the 229 patients died from myocardial infarction within 12 weeks of admission. The results of the study indicated that the patients who died had been in ward situations inappropriate to their locus of control—that is, patients either with an internal locus of control who ended up in the low-participation group or those with an external locus of control who ended up in the high-participation group. In this case, the ability of patients to use certain kinds of information (i.e., effective self-help techniques) depended on their locus of control.

The study also found that if patients were given considerable information about their medical conditions but not provided the opportunity to assist in their own recovery or to divert themselves (with visitors, magazines, television, and so on), then long hospital stays resulted. Therefore, it is suggested that if medical information is provided to a patient, some degree of participation or at least the opportunity for distraction should also be provided.

In sum, the locus of control dimension provides information about an individual's style of dealing with life; some individuals may behave as if they are calling the shots, whereas others may behave as if fate, chance, or other people are primarily responsible for what happens to them. Depending on the circumstances, such styles may or may not be adaptive; patients with an external locus of control might, for example, do very poorly in a rehabilitation situation yet do quite well in an intensive care unit where they are kept relatively immobilized. Overall, the research to date suggests that assessment of the locus of control dimension in patients can provide information useful for effective medical care.

REPRESSION-SENSITIZATION

Repression, according to psychoanalytic theory, is the exclusion from awareness by the unconscious of certain threatening conflicts or perceptions. The repression-sensitization personality dimension is based on somewhat the same notion, although it is specifically geared to stimulus perception. Basically, individuals characterized as *repressors* are those who have a high threshold for perceiving stimuli; for these people, stimuli have to be intense or to last a long time to be perceived. Those characterized as *sensitizers*, on the other hand, have a lower threshold for perceiving stimuli (Gordon, 1957). Both repressors and sensitizers are thought to have developed general coping styles related to the behavior in question. Sensitizers tend to seek out information as a way of preparing for a stressful situation, whereas repressors tend to ignore or avoid information.

Measurement of the dimension of repression-sensitization is accomplished by means of an objective self-report scale, much like the locus-of-control scale described earlier. A scale developed by Byrne (1964) and a more recent adaptation of same (Epstein and Fenz, 1967) are those most commonly used today.

The coping styles of individuals characterized as repressors or sensitizers have, as you might guess, a significant impact on their health care. A repressor will tend to ignore symptoms and to discount any information provided, whereas a sensitizer will actively attempt to learn more about symptoms and eagerly request medical advice. Some knowledge of the repression-sensitization dimension may thus be useful in certain types of medical intervention. The reader may recall from the previous chapter that cognitive changes can be effected by describing to patients what sensations and other experiences will occur during medical procedures. Shipley, Butt, and Horowitz (1979) examined a method designed to alleviate anxiety in which patients were informed in advance about the experience they would have during a stressful endoscopy examination. Specifically, the patients were shown an explicit endoscopy on videotape. The effectiveness of this procedure was determined afterwards through measurements of heart rate during the actual endoscopy, through physician-nurse anxiety ratings, and through self-report. In general, it was discovered that the showing of the videotape effectively reduced anxiety in those individuals classified as sensitizers, whereas certain measures of anxiety such as heart rate increased in those classified as repressors.

In sum, the primary current application of the repression-sensitization dimension in medical practice occurs in the context of providing effective preparation for medical procedures. Along with information derived from the internal-external locus of control dimension, the repression-sensitization dimension can be used to identify the most effective health care procedures for any given patient.

TYPE A PERSONALITY

The *Type A personality* is one that exhibits a cluster of behaviors associated with increased risk of heart disease. This behavior pattern was described by Friedman and Rosenman (1974) as "an action-emotion complex that can be observed in any person who is aggressively involved in a chronic, incessant struggle to achieve more and more in less and less time, and if required to do so, against the opposing effects of other persons and things" and by Glass (1977) as "competitive achievement striving, a sense of time urgency, and hostility" (p. 178). The Type A personality has also been described as including the following characteristics (Matteson and Ivancevich, 1980; Suinn, 1977):

(a) a constant sense of time urgency
(b) striving to accomplish more in less and less time
(c) a competitive and driving attitude
(d) hostility that is easily provoked, either overtly or covertly
(e) chronic impatience
(f) discomfort during inactivity or relaxation
(g) an overemphasis on actual accomplishment with a depreciation of experiencing or feeling

In simple terms, the individual with a Type A personality tends to be fiercely competitive and will generally put out the maximum effort even when a given task does not require it. Such persons can often be identified by their competitive attitudes in "friendly" games of sports and can be described in this connection and others as almost "doomed to success." Indeed, they typically rise to the tops of their profession due to their capacity for hard work and their persistence. Such a pattern of behavior is actually quite common among health care professionals, because the long hours, competition, and time pressures associated with medical, nursing, and graduate schools tend to select for precisely those Type A qualities.

Unfortunately, individuals identified as Type A personalities have more than twice the rate of heart disease as those who do not exhibit this pattern of behavior (Rosenman et al., 1975). Furthermore, this risk persists even when conventional risk factors (such as alcohol intake and smoking) are controlled for (Orth-Gomer, Ahlborn, and Theorell, 1980).

Measurement of Type A personality is most often accomplished by means of the Jenkins Activity Survey (Jenkins, Zyzanski, and Rosenman, 1979), a multiple-choice questionnaire that requires individuals to respond to examples of a variety of situations. It includes questions such as "How would your wife (or closest friend) rate you?"

and "Do you ever set deadlines or quotas for yourself at work or at home?" Answers consistent with Type A personality would include the choices "Definitely hard-driving and competitive" and "Yes, once a week or more often." High scores on this test are interpreted as fitting the Type A behavior pattern.

Can anything be done about the Type A pattern? Some would say that it might not be beneficial to change a behavior pattern that generally results in success. A number of clinicians, however, have attempted to teach individuals with Type A personality to develop relaxation coping techniques so that they might deal with particularly stressful situations in more effective ways (Roskies et al., 1978, 1979; Suinn, 1974). The theory behind the relaxation approach is that, when relaxed, one cannot simultaneously be tense and anxious. Thus, if an individual learns to relax in the face of stressors, he or she will not react with tension at the same time. Theoretically, it is the constant response of tension and anxiety to stressful situations that leads to the increased risk of coronary heart disease. (See Bieliauskas, 1982, for a further discussion of Type A behavior and stress.)

In sum, each of the independent personality dimensions discussed in this chapter describes a particular aspect of health-related behaviors rather than providing a comprehensive overview or an attempt to systematize all behaviors. The augmenter-reducer dimension concentrates on symptom perception, whereas the internal-external locus of control dimension focuses on the individual's responses to illness and treatment. The repression-sensitization dimension focuses on symptom action, whereas the Type A personality dimension concentrates on a particular kind of symptom formation. Each of these approaches is supported by evidence in the particular area it addresses, although none of them proposes to be a general explanation for health-related behaviors. Thus, the health care practitioner must take a "multiple-choice" approach geared to finding and employing the most useful concept for the particular behavior he or she is studying. Although a unified theory of personality would offer a more comprehensive perspective on individual behavior, the demonstrated success of the independent perspectives on individual behavior suggests that a truly unified theory of behavior is yet to be created.

INDIVIDUAL
DIFFERENCES
AND INTELLIGENCE

At first glance, *intelligence* might not seem to be an organizing concept for behavior in the sense that other personality theories or concepts are. However, this more likely reflects a misconception about intelligence than a lack of relevance in the concept. What is meant by intelligence? Some would suggest that no definition at all is required because all intelligent people know what intelligence is: "it is the thing that the other guy lacks" (McNemar, 1964, p. 871).

More seriously, however, intelligence has historically been looked upon as a sort of general index of mental functioning, a measure of the ability to learn, to abstract, and to profit from experience. The concept of intelligence thus also describes the degree of flexibility or versatility exhibited by the individual; in still more contemporary terms, we might define intelligence as the ability to adjust and to achieve. Accordingly, intelligence, as measured by tests, is often used as an indicator for school placement, vocational guidance, job placement, and so on.

As an index of mental functioning, intelligence was previously thought to pervade all tasks performed by an individual and all of that individual's abilities. It was seen as a general factor, the factor g (Spearman, 1927); this factor "far from being confined to some small set of abilities . . . may enter into all abilities whatsoever" (p. 77). However, given that g was considered such an overriding factor, the argument was easily made that it represented some kind of native, innate ability; each individual was therefore believed to have an inborn quantity of this g, or intelligence. Needless to say, there was considerable outcry at such a notion, particularly in the United States, a nation that believes all are created equal.

A number of researchers subsequently attempted to define intelligence as only one representation of an individual's abilities. They proposed that, in reality, each of us has several different kinds of intelligence; whereas one individual might be intelligent in one area, a second individual might be intelligent in another. In short, each of us was seen as possessing certain "gifts." In this connection, Guilford (1959) and Getzels and Jackson (1969) described certain dimensions of intellect, including creativity, memory, divergent thinking, and so on. They argued that, in much of our school system, these individual talents are often ignored with respect to the development of potential in individual students. Although this approach was popular in the 1950s and 1960s, little utility has come of it. McNemar (1964) pointed out that if we attempt to statistically remove the intelligence (g) factor from performance levels on a wide variety of different tasks, we will find it cannot be done. In fact, the g factor fares as well as or better than "creativity" or other factors reflecting "gifts" in predicting abilities such as school performance. Rather, claims McNemar, the tests of such "gifts" in fact are measuring the same thing that general intelligence tests measure, but are only giving new names to an older concept.

Despite the attacks leveled at the approach, intelligence, as measured by tests, does correlate well with school grades and various achievement criteria. These correlations, however, become stronger (to a point) as an individual becomes older; therefore, the correlation between a criterion such as school performance and measured intelligence will be lower in a young child than in a teenager.

A more reasonable way to view intelligence, one that takes into account its utility as a concept but perhaps does not provoke the reaction that a "mental functioning index" view would, is to see it as "the tendency for each organism to process all kinds of information at a similar level of efficiency" (Lezak, 1976, p. 15). From this point of view, intelligence becomes a measure of overall ability to perform at about the same level on a variety of different intellectual tasks (McNemar, 1964). As it happens, for the popular view that an individual could be strong in one area ("gifted") while weak in others, "there was found no support whatever. On the contrary, it appeared

FIGURE 7. A three-stage hierarchy. (Humphreys, 1962; appearing in Lezak, 1976, Figure 2.1, p. 17. Reprinted by permission of the American Psychological Association, Oxford Press, and the author.)

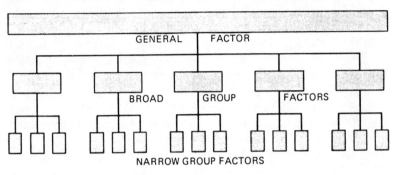

that any failure in anything is rather a bad than a good augury for other things" (Spearman and Jones, 1950, p.7).

In what way, then, do specific abilities relate to more general abilities? According to Lezak (1976, p. 16), "factor analytic studies of intellectual behavior have consistently demonstrated a hierarchical organization of mental abilities." Figure 7 illustrates such a hierarchical organization. At the top is the general factor g. Below that are the broad group factors, representing "broad classes of mental abilities such as verbal, computational, or visual organization" (Lezak, 1976, p. 17). Further down are the narrow group factors, which refer to more specific abilities such as mathematical skill.

The testing of any given factor measures only a narrow range of abilities, and the broader factor is inferred. The wider the range in which tests are given, the safer would be the inference to the broader factor. Thus, a test of skill in differential calculus would suggest an inference of good computing abilities. Further tests of skill in integral calculus, logarithmic functions, and so on, if scored the same way, would yield even more confidence in the inference relating to computational facility. That is, inference to the general factor becomes more valid as more different kinds of narrow measures are applied. Thus, we might want to give tests of verbal and spatially related narrow skills in addition to computational tests to abstract the measurement of the general factor g.

MEASUREMENT OF INTELLIGENCE

Alfred Binet was commissioned in 1904 by the Minister of Public Instruction in France to devise a method for detecting children who were "subnormal" in intellectual abilities so that they could be placed in special schools. Binet came up with a test in which the tasks and problems were appropriate to a given child's age. He determined this age factor by examining a number of children and estimating the quantity of particular items a child of a given age should be able to answer successfully; *norms,* or expected performances, were thus established. A large number of items, which tapped a large number of different abilities, were employed: children were asked to perform tasks ranging from drawing figures to computing mathematical problems to remembering stimuli. In line with the definition of intelligence, the test was designed to measure a potential or tendency rather than a particular skill in any single area. In fact, the test attempted to measure a general ability to perform a number of different tasks. Furthermore, the number of questions answered correctly by most children at a given age was established as a norm for a *mental age.* Thus, if most seven-year-old children correctly answered 20 items, then the correct answering of 20 items represented a mental age of seven in any given individual (Binet and Simon, 1915).

However, mental age is not a stable measure. Every child learns over time and thus can later answer a larger number of items correctly. To create a more stable reference that better described intellectual ability, Stern (1914) proposed that the measured mental age be divided by the chronological age of the child to give an *intellectual quotient* (IQ); this quotient appeared to be quite stable. The formula for the IQ took this form:

$$\frac{\text{Mental Age}}{\text{Chronological Age}} \times 100 = \text{Intelligence Quotient}$$

The quotient is multiplied by one hundred to get rid of the decimals and to make it more readable. Thus, a child of eight years who correctly answers the number of items appropriate for an eight-year-old would score an IQ of 100 (8/8 × 100 = 100). One hundred thus becomes the average IQ score. On the other hand, a child of six who correctly answers the same number of items appropriate for a nine-year-old would score an IQ of 150.

Terman (1916) from Stanford University adapted the Binet test for an American population; this adaptation is in wide use today and is known as the Stanford-Binet Intelligence Scale (Terman and Merrill, 1973). However, although the test is applicable to young adults up to the age of eighteen, determination of the IQ by the mental and chronological age method becomes less accurate once a stable level of learning has been achieved. Therefore, as one peaks in terms of learning ability (that is, one does not gain the ability to do greater number of items and thus increase "mental age"), the ratio of mental age to chronological age gets smaller as age increases. This does not mean that intelligence decreases, only that the method for computing it is no longer accurate.

In addition, although the Stanford-Binet test assesses a number of different abilities, there is no breakdown of the areas being examined; for this reason, no "broad group factors" can be derived from the test scores. These factors, however, are frequently of value in determining whether a test subject has a specific difficulty or is demonstrating a low "g" factor. Therefore, the Stanford-Binet test is generally restricted to children between two and five years of age; for those older than five, intelligence is computed by means of the *deviation IQ*, which is derived from a standard statistical distribution of scores on a variety of test items and thus provides a categorical breakdown of the abilities being tested.

The Wechsler Scales, now the most popular test for the measurement of intelligence, are based on the deviation IQ. They consist of items that are broken down into large categories—verbal scales and performance scales. In general, the verbal scales concentrate on tasks that measure skills requiring the use of language, whereas the performance scales measure motor dexterity and visual-spatial skills. Each set of scales is composed of a number of subtests measuring different aspects of verbal or performance abilities.

Please refer now to Figure 8 as we discuss the derivation of scores on the Wechsler Scales. The scores achieved on each subtest are first converted to standard scores. Each standard score is equivalent to the average (mean) score of a group of individuals taking the subtest in question; this average is set at a given number so that scores above

FIGURE 8. A normal distribution (or bell-shaped curve). Many psychological characteristics, such as intelligence, are found to be normally distributed in the population at large. This fact facilitates rapid and precise communication about test scores. For example, one can report a *percentile equivalent*, which represents the proportion of individual scores in a group that are less than or equal to a given score in the population at large. A standard score indicates how far a score is from the average (or mean) score; thus a standard score of +2 is considerably *above* the mean, and one of −2 is exactly the same distance *below* the mean. (From *Psychology Today: An Introduction,* 1972, Figure 20.8, p. 395. Reprinted by permission of Random House, Inc.)

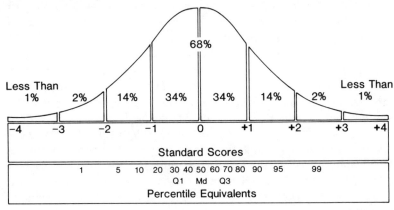

or below it can be computed on the basis of how far the scores are from the average. The resulting figures are expressed as *standard deviations,* which represent the percentages of individuals who achieved particular scores. In Figure 8, the mean score on a test is arbitrarily set at zero; approximately one-third (34 percent) of those scoring above the average and one-third of those scoring below are within one standard deviation, the standard scores here being +1 and −1 for the limits of these percentages. The next 14 percent above and below the average comprise the second standard deviation, and standard scores of +2 and −2 are assigned to the limits of these percentages. At this point, we have accounted for 96 percent of the individuals taking the test. The next 2 percent above and below the average comprise the third standard deviation, which now accounts for almost all of the individuals taking the test. Computations for actual standard scores and standard deviations are, of course, more complex than Figure 8 would seem to indicate. Further descriptions of such calculations can be found in any standard statistical text (e.g., Downie and Heath, 1965). Similarly, one can interpret a distribution of scores on a test in terms of *percentile equivalent*, which refers to the proportion of scores that are less than or equal to the score one is interested in.

Standard scores are used for tests for the purpose of making comparisons. How can we equate an arithmetic test with a vocabulary test if they measure different skills and probably differ in the number of items? A score of 8 items correct on one test and the same score on another test may reflect entirely different abilities if one test has 10 items and the other has 20 items. However, if we calculate that 90 percent of the individuals in a group achieved a score of 8 out of 10 items correct while on another test 90 percent achieved a score of 16 out of 20, that permits us to compare one test with the other; we can also conclude, for instance, that a given individual scoring 80 percent on the first test had only an average score, whereas an individual scoring 80 percent correct on the second test achieved a very good score compared to the rest of the group. In terms of standard scores, the first individual would get a score of about 0 on the first test and a score of about +2 on the second test.

The subtests on the Wechsler Scales are converted into standard scores for all individuals taking the test at the time the tests were normed, that is, administered to large groups. Each subtest is then arbitrarily assigned an average value of 10 with a standard deviation of 3 (in Figure 8, a score of 10 would fall at a standard score of +1, and a score of 7 would fall at a standard score of −1). Once standard scores for each subtest are obtained, they are added together (since they are now comparable); the totals on the verbal scales obtain a verbal score and the totals on the performance scales obtain a performance score. At this point, the scores are converted into intelligence quotients (IQs). The sum of standard scores is compared to the standard scores obtained in a given age group (for example all 16- and 17-year-olds). The distribution of standard scores for all in a given age group approximates the distribution seen in Figure 8, and the average IQ is arbitrarily set at 100, with standard deviations of 15. Thus, an individual who obtains a sum of verbal scores equal to or greater than 84 percent of his or her relative group would receive an IQ of 115. (In Figure 8, this percentage would include all who scored less than the standard score of +1, as seen at the center and on the left side of the figure.) Since this IQ is based on standard deviations in a normal distribution of scores, it is called a deviation IQ. In the case of the Wechsler Scales, an individual would thus receive a verbal IQ (from a comparison with the sum of standard verbal scores), a performance IQ (from a comparison with the sum of all standard performance scores) and a full scale IQ (from comparisons with the sum of all standard scores). Since these scores are always compared to those achieved in a relative age group, the individual's IQ will not decrease over time as would be the case with the Stanford-Binet calculation.

As already noted, the comparison groups for the Wechsler Scales include all individuals of a given age. These comparison groups were composed, at the time the tests were constructed, on the basis of sex, race, and ethnic ratios representative of the average population of the United States for each age. The tests have been revised a number of times as the population of the United States has changed, and the references cited for the tests are the most recent. We could, of course, identify IQ scores relative to any group of our choice—for example, relative to all engineers, all swimmers, all college students, or all medical students. In the case of the Wechsler Scales, however, the comparison group is a representative sample of all individuals in the United States in a given age bracket.

The Wechsler Scales are geared to three overall age groups. The scale for young children, the Wechsler Preschool and Primary Scale of Intelligence (WPPSI), is designed for children from four to six and one-half years of age (Wechsler, 1967). The Wechsler Intelligence Scale for Children-Revised (WISC-R) is designed for children aged six to sixteen years, eleven months (Wechsler, 1974). The Wechsler Adult Intelligence Scale-Revised (WAIS-R) is designed for adults aged sixteen years and older (Wechsler, 1981).

As already mentioned, the Wechsler Scales are the most popular in use today, and the IQs reported on the basis of these tests are generally expressed in terms of performance, verbal, and full scale scores. These tests provide a good estimate of an individual's overall intellectual abilities. As you might guess, the interpretation of verbal scores versus performance scores and of individual subtest scores has been attempted by many researchers. Although many useful findings have been reported, there is still considerable controversy over the

Table 1. Wechsler's Intelligence Classifications

IQ	Classification	Per Cent Included
130 and above	Very Superior	2.2
120 - 129	Superior	6.7
110 - 119	Bright Normal	16.1
90 - 109	Average	50.0
80 - 89	Dull Normal	16.1
70 - 79	Borderline	6.7
69 and below	Mental Defective	2.2

question of how the various scores relate to each other in terms of personality variables. Further discussion of these matters is not possible in this volume, but a good reference for the interested reader is Matarazzo (1972).

What do IQ scores mean in practical terms? More specifically, what is meant when an IQ score is used to designate someone as mentally retarded or intellectually superior? Such designations in Wechsler's terms would be expressed statistically. Referring again to the percentages in Figure 8, we can interpret the designations of Wechsler in Table 1 as a distribution of scores. An IQ between 90 and 109 represents 50 percent of the population in question and is termed "average." The scores above and below are similarly representative of percentages of the population above and below the average range.

The upper levels of IQ are not difficult to interpret. It is generally believed that an individual must have an IQ of 100 to be successful in college and an IQ of 120 or better to be successful in graduate or professional schools. In general, the higher the better. But what about the lower levels? The implications of low scores are debatable, but a summary of generally accepted categories is given in Tables 2 and 3. The designations for IQ scores in these tables—such as mild, moderate, and profound retardation—are somewhat arbitrary, although they do represent the standard nomenclature. The true

87

Table 2. Capacities and Limitations of Mentally Retarded Adults

Capacities	Limitations
Mild Retardation: IQ from 51 to 70 *(Adult Mental Ages of 7 to 12 Years)*	
Can perform routine factory or farm work. Can learn to read and write. Can evolve into self-supporting citizens under favorable environment.	Do not usually progress past five to six years of schooling. Often incapable of recognizing their moral and legal obligations and therefore apt to become delinquents, prostitutes, and petty thieves when not properly guided. Their physical maturity, in the absence of corresponding mental maturity, predisposes to unregulated and sometimes antisocial behavior.
Moderate to Severe Retardation: IQ from 26 to 50 *(Adult Mental Ages of 3 to 7 Years)*	
Can learn to talk. Can do simple work under supervision, such as mopping floors, rough painting, digging, and simple farm chores. If tractable and closely supervised, may possibly be self-supporting.	Usually do not understand the value of money. Usually should not be permitted to live outside of institutions or away from very close supervision of the families. May be dangerous to self or others when emotionally upset or sexually aroused.
Severe to Profound Retardation: IQ up to 25 *(Adult Mental Age of 2 Years)*	
May learn to eat food without aid. May make themselves understood by grunts or even a few simple words. May learn to dress themselves partially.	Must be institutionalized to avoid common dangers of life. Often have poor physical stamina and are subject to early demise. Usually unable to contribute constructively in any task and require constant supervision.

(From Kahn & Giffen, pp. 56-57. Reprinted by permission of Pergamon Press and the authors.)

meaning of the IQ scores is better represented by the behavioral implications associated with them.

There are numerous scales other than Wechsler's used to measure intelligence. I will mention only one here, since it is commonly used in health care settings—the Peabody Picture Vocabulary Test (Dunn, 1959). This test is popular because it is shorter and easier to administer than the Wechsler Scales (about 10 minutes versus about 60 to 90 minutes). Its IQ scores are also determined by the standard deviation method, and they generally compare well with Wechsler Scale IQ scores. However, the Peabody test scores are based entirely on verbal comprehension abilities (understanding

Table 3. Levels of Adaptive Behavior

Level	Preschool Age 0-5 Maturation and Development	School Age 6-21 Training and Education	Adult 21 Social and Vocational Adequacy
Mild	Can develop social and communication skills; minimal retardation in sensorimotor areas; rarely distinguished from normal until later age.	Can learn academic skills to approximately 6th grade level by late teens. Cannot learn general high school subjects. Needs special education, particularly at secondary school age levels.	Capable of social and vocational adequacy with proper education and training. Frequently needs supervision and guidance when under serious social or economic stress.
Moderate	Can talk or learn to communicate; poor social awareness; fair motor development; may profit from self-help; can be managed with moderate supervision.	Can learn functional academic skills to approximately 4th grade level by late teens if given special education.	Capable of self-maintenance in unskilled or semi-skilled occupations; needs supervision and guidance when under mild social or economic stress.
Severe	Poor motor development; speech is minimal, generally unable to profit from training in self-help; little or no communication skills.	Can talk or learn to communicate; can be trained in elemental health habits; cannot learn functional academic skills; profits from systematic habit training.	Can contribute partially to self-support under complete supervision; can develop self-protection skills to a minimal useful level in controlled environment.
Profound	Gross retardation; minimal capacity for functioning in sensorimotor areas; needs nursing care.	Some motor development present; cannot profit from training in self-help; needs total care.	Some motor and speech development; totally incapable of self-maintenance; needs complete care and supervision.

(From Sloan & Birch, 1955, p. 262. Reprinted by permission of the American Association on Mental Deficiency and the authors.)

what words mean) and do not consider other abilities in the measurement of intelligence. Certain individuals may thus be at a disadvantage with such a test. In addition, research has indicated that Peabody test scores tend to be slightly higher than Wechsler scores for the same individual.

As a final note on measurement, I will add that intelligence tests should not be confused with achievement tests. Intelligence tests are designed to measure an individual's potential, whereas achievement tests are designed to measure what an individual actually knows in a given area. The later tests are thus used to assess general accomplishment in school, the effectiveness of a training program, and so on. The most commonly used achievement tests are those designed for

89

school-aged children and are often employed to assess learning difficulties. The Wide Range Achievement Test (WRAT) (Jastak and Jastak, 1965) and the Peabody Individual Achievement Test (PIAT) (Dunn and Markwardt, 1970) are those that the health care professional is most likely to encounter. These tests measure abilities in reading, spelling, arithmetic, and so on—in other words, basic learning skills. They are generally designed for children five to eighteen years of age, and they provide scores that can be interpreted relative to a child's general age group or school grade group.

IMPLICATIONS FOR HEALTH CARE

Now that we have discussed the structure of intelligence tests and what they measure when an IQ score is reported, we must determine the application of this information to health care. In general, the IQ score gives a judgment of an individual's general potential. Because of the nature of how IQ tests are constructed, based primarily on intellectual processing items, behaviors they predict the best are academically related. Thus, the correlation between the IQ scores and school grades is approximately .50 (by squaring the correlation one sees how much of the variance in one variable is predicted by another; the correlation of .50 means that IQ scores predict approximately 25 percent of the variability in school grades). Correlations between IQ scores and success in personal service jobs are about .61. In less academically related variables, the predictions are lower; correlations between IQ scores and job training performance are about .38 while correlations between IQ scores and success at manual labor are about 0 (Krech and Crutchfield, 1965). In general, the more complex the understanding of concepts, principles, or technical relationships which is required for a given behavior, the more predictive is the IQ score for the ability to perform the behavior successfully.

Perhaps the most obvious application of the estimate of intelligence occurs in direct communication with patients, who necessarily must understand what they are told about the illness they are experiencing and the purpose of the medical procedures they will undergo. It is not uncommon for a health care professional to explain an illness or a particular procedure to a patient who does not comprehend what has been said. This is the fault not of the patient but of the professional who fails to consider the patient's situation. With some effort, it really is possible to explain medical concepts and procedures in a way that makes sense to the patient. It should also be kept in mind that a patient's level of understanding is not necessarily a function of intelligence. Indeed, medical explanations laced with jargon and technical terms would be incomprehensible to *anyone* unfamiliar with the medical field, quite regardless of the intelligence factor. Overall, the attempt to speak to patients in understandable terms always serves the best interests of both the practitioner and the patient.

Another mistake to be avoided is the assumption of low intelligence, with a consequent patronizing of the patient in question. We all know of health practitioners who refrain from explaining anything because they feel that the patient "wouldn't understand." On one occasion, for instance, I was called to see an in-patient who had developed cerebrospinal rhinorrhea subsequent to a skull fracture. The patient had also developed meningitis and was slightly delirious. I was called because the patient was behaving in a hostile way towards the hospital staff, refusing to listen to instructions, and becoming difficult to control. He appeared to me to be of lower socioeconomic status; his clothes were shabby and he had not shaved for several days. The records indicated that he worked as a general construction laborer.

It was evident that the hospital staff had assumed this patient to be of low intelligence; little was explained to him, staff members talked about him in his room in the mistaken belief that he couldn't understand what was being said, and his questions were seldom given answers other than the assurance that everything being done was "for his own good." On testing, however, the patient scored an IQ of 130 (that is, in the very superior range). The patient complained that he couldn't figure out what was going on; he knew he was feeling poorly but didn't know why, and he didn't understand the purpose of the medications he was taking or why various procedures were being performed. Following my report to the staff of this patient's capacities and of the mistreatment he felt he'd received, the staff took a more respectful attitude, explained matters to him clearly, and consulted him or recommended procedures. Although the patient was still quite ill, his disruptive behavior ceased and effective hospital care was resumed.

Whatever its source, whatever its background, intelligence is a concept that describes the general capacity of the individual to engage in a wide variety of tasks. It can be measured in a meaningful way. In the health care field, intelligence pertains to how well the professional can explain necessary procedures, concepts, and regimens to a patient and what complex behaviors can be expected on the part of the patient. It also is important in insuring that patients are given adequate information about their health care. It will have an effect on how a patient perceives his or her symptoms and the intellectual resources available to a patient to engage in effective action about the symptoms. Intelligence relates to the variety, complexity, and flexibility of behaviors formed in one's personality.

ASSESSMENT METHODS

We have now covered many of the existing approaches to understanding individual human behavior. In this chapter, we will discuss certain methods of assessing behavior in terms of the data appropriate to the approach we wish to employ. Basically, there are three general methods for personality assessment: interviewing, psychological testing, and behavioral rating or sampling.

THE INTERVIEW

In the interview situations, the health care professional is basically concerned with obtaining information about an individual, arrived at by asking questions and acquiring answers, either explicitly or implicitly. The professional can ask the person directly or ask someone who knows the person. One such question might be "Does coming into the hospital make you feel anxious?" or, more generally, "What things are happening in your life that make your symptoms worse?" It is surprising to find how often patients will respond with forthright answers, so long as the questions are asked in a sensitive manner and in a way that appears relevant to the patient. Most patients are willing to discuss such matters as physical symptoms that cause emotional distress and emotional distress that causes or exacerbates physical symptoms. But a patient will balk at questions perceived as prying and irrelevant, as well as questions suggesting that the professional does not believe the patient's symptoms are real. It is best to keep in mind that *all* symptoms are real to the patient and that the purpose of the interviews is effective patient care rather than an opportunity to prove something. If a patient perceives this effort at sensitivity, he or she is likely to cooperate willingly by answering questions.

Korchin (1976, p. 169) summarized the types of data on personality that can be obtained in the interview:

(1) statements by the patient himself, describing characteristic feelings of his current and past life ("I have always been shy with girls"); (2) accompanying behaviors, some unintended and outside of awareness (e.g., tremulous voice); and (3) reactions inspired by the clinician, whether based on real or fantasied acts (e.g., annoyance at a seemingly unsympathetic response). The difficult task of the clinician is to note and remember the content of the patient's utterances, observe his behavior, and assess the contribution of his own actions to what he hears and sees. It is a task which requires considerable skill, sensitivity, and flexibility.

Korchin (1976) also discussed the format of the interview as consisting of three stages. It is helpful to keep these stages in mind because their neglect may result in upsetting the patient at the least and in obtaining incomplete and erroneous information at the worst. The first stage is the *opening phase*. At this point, at least a few minutes should be spent in making the patient comfortable and in establishing some kind of relationship. For any relationship to take place, the health care professional must introduce him or herself, clarify his or her role in the patient's care, and explain the purpose of the questions to be asked. The patient should always be permitted – indeed, encouraged – to ask questions about any matters not understood. As Korchin further noted, "Particularly at the outset . . . questions are few and brief, and intended mainly to encourage the patient to develop themes relevant to him in his own fashion. Particular comments may pique our curiosity, but it is well to hold off any inquiry in depth until the patient has ranged freely over matters most urgent and important to him" (p. 177). It is crucial, at this stage, that the patient senses some understanding on the professional's part of the problem itself and how it is being experienced. Thus, it is important to allow the patient to describe the problem in his or her own words.

In the second phase, the *middle portion*, information is obtained that will help the health care professional to formulate at least a tentative hypothesis about the patient's symptoms. Occurrence of stressing life experiences, strained family relationships, the patient's typical reactions to illness—these are all important matters to be clarified. As a rule of thumb, the professional should determine what impact the illness is having on the patient's work, social and family relationships, recreational activities, and sexual behavior. In the process, the professional can decide whether reinforcers are present that behaviorally exaggerate certain symptoms and whether concerns external to the patient's illness are significantly contributing to the observed distress.

It is also during this middle portion of the interview that the professional must choose the particular approach to be used. If an analytic approach is the most appropriate in a given case, defense mechanisms, likely routes for impulse expression, and the nature of particular conflicts will be explored. If on the other hand a behavioral approach seems more relevant, a concentration on conditional stimuli, reinforcers, and responses will be in order. Then again, it is also possible to apply more than one approach, depending on the circumstances of the patient (as will be further discussed in the next chapter). In this case, information-gathering must pertain specifically to those portions of the approaches the professional wishes to adopt. For example, the professional might identify particular dependency needs in a patient and then explore aspects of the patient's illness that serve as reinforcers for dependent-related behaviors.

At all times during the interview, the professional must pay close attention to the patient's nonverbal behavior. This cautionary note may seem overstated but then it is surprising how often health care professionals fail to notice the pained facial expression, the wringing of hands, or the restless shifting of the body as a patient explains that he feels fine and that he has no psychological concerns. It is also important to be sensitive to incongruencies of emotion or expression during a patient's description of the impact of symptoms on his or her daily life. An example of such incongruence is the classic diagnostic feature *la belle indifference*, which occurs in the presence of conversion reaction (see Chapter 2) and refers to the amazing lack of distress or concern exhibited by a patient who is describing a severely disabling symptom such as paralysis of a limb. When such an incongruence is noted, the professional should at least be alerted to the possibility that some serious underlying issue is present relating to the topic under discussion.

To ensure that the information acquired from a patient is comprehensive, a professional might employ a *structured interview* consisting of a list of standard questions that call for either specific (multiple choice) or open-ended answers. By means of such interviews, patients can be compared with each other or with themselves at different points in time. Also available to the professional are the structured interviews known as *rating scales,* in which specific patient characteristics are detailed and then rated along several dimensions; in this interview format, the questions are not specified, but the content to be reviewed is.

One notable example of a structured interview is the type developed to measure Type A (coronary prone) patterns of behavior (Rosenman, 1978), which predates the popular Jenkins Activity Survey mentioned in Chapter 6. Another popular interview format, designed to assess more pathological patterns of behavior but also useful in general personality description, is the Schedule for Affective Disorders and Schizophrenia (SADS) (Spitzer and Endicott, 1978). By this method, a wide range of information can be gathered for the purpose of psychiatric assessment.

Examples of rating scales, on the other hand, include the Inpatient Multidimensional Psychiatric Scale (IMPS) (Lorr, McNair, Klett, and Lasky, 1966) and the Hamilton Psychiatric Rating Scale for Depression (Hamilton, 1967). These scales basically list a number of specific behaviors, attitudes, and perceptions, which are then checked for each patient and rated along a continuum from "not present" to "significantly present." A score is then obtained by summing the ratings along several dimensions. In contrast to the specific questions associated with structured interviews, the rating scales require the examiner to assign ratings to predetermined behaviors. The strengths and weaknesses of the rating scales are similar to those for structured interviews.

A number of other similar methods are available, all having the express purpose of providing a reliable and complete information base for describing patients. The disadvantage of such methods, however, is that they can take a great deal of time to administer and, if used in entirety, may obtain information that is not always of interest. Nevertheless, for the interviewer in need of information that must be compared over time, or between patients, the structured interview format is far superior to open-ended interviews.

The main objective in the third phase of the interview, called the *final phase,* is "to restore the patient's calm, give him information, and plan with him the next steps" (Korchin, 1976, p. 180). At this time, an understanding and concern for the patient should be communicated, along with a realistic appraisal of the patient's situation. The patient should be given neither blanket reassurance nor a void of information; rather, the professional should express empathy with the patient and provide preliminary opinions and likely plans for proceeding from that point.

PSYCHOLOGICAL TESTING

Following the interview, the professional may find it desirable to obtain a sample of the patient's behavior, either by measuring the patient's response in unusual situations or by giving the patient questions with limited response choices so that they can be compared to the responses of patients with known characteristics. In brief, such psychological testing is a short-cut to getting to know a person better. If the professional had known a given patient for a lengthy period of time and thus had the background to evaluate that patient's behavior, testing would not be necessary. But hospital stays are typically brief and frequently demand an assessment of personality organization that goes beyond the interview but is constrained by time. Psychological testing fulfills this purpose.

Objective Tests

There are basically two types of psychological tests, *objective* and *projective.* Objective tests provide fixed questions (stimuli) and permit fixed responses. With this type of test, the professional can compare specific patient responses to those of other patients with known characteristics. The Wechsler Scales mentioned in the previous chapter are objective tests; here, too, specific questions are asked, only certain answers are permitted for scoring purposes, and the responses can be compared to those obtained from other groups.

Much like the intelligence tests, objective tests for personality assessment are primarily *self-report inventories.* These inventories are composed of questions that a patient answers, generally in a "true-false" or multiple-choice fashion. The most popular self-report inventory in use today is the Minnesota Multiphasic Personality Inventory

97

(MMPI) (Hathaway and McKinley, 1943). This test contains 566 items, each of which is marked as "true" or "false" as it applies to the person taking the test. The items chosen for this test were actuarially determined; that is, they were selected not because of the specific characteristics they revealed but because certain groups of people had previously answered them in a particular way. These groups, for the most part, are comprised of patients with a particular psychiatric diagnosis. The answers provided by these groups are compared to the answers given by a "normal" group of test-takers. In general, the more items an individual answers in the same way as answered by a particular diagnosed group, the more characteristics this individual is believed to share with that group.

The reader may wonder why a test designed for measuring responses based on psychiatric illness would be used for general personality assessment. As previously mentioned, test items answered in a particular way indicate specific characteristics of behavior, those characteristics shared by the group in which an individual is compared. These characteristics, in turn, can reveal significant information about personality organization. For example, one of the clinical scales included on the MMPI is called "conversion hysteria." The referent for the items on this scale was a group of patients with this diagnosis. As noted in Chapter 2, one of the main features of this psychiatric condition is a failure to directly express an unacceptable impulse, with a somatic symptom utilized instead by way of indirect expression. The defense mechanism operating here is repression, the act of unconsciously keeping the impulse from awareness. The higher the score on the Conversion Hysteria Scale, the greater is the individual's repression as a psychological defense. Personality assessment by means of the other MMPI scales proceeds along the same lines.

Altogether, the MMPI has three validity scales and ten clinical scales. The validity scales measure those dimensions of test taking that suggest whether or not the subject is giving honest, truthful, and valid answers. The MMPI thus provides an index of lying, understating, or exaggerating. The validity scales also provide an index by which the clinical scales are to be interpreted. These latter scales break down as follows:

(a) Hypochondriasis
(b) Depression

(c) Conversion Hysteria
(d) Psychopathic Deviancy
(e) Masculinity/Femininity
(f) Paranoia
(g) Psychasthenia (anxiety/distress)
(h) Schizophrenia
(i) Hypomania
(j) Social Introversion (a tendency to withdraw or to isolate oneself)

The MMPI is routinely used in medical practice to assess behavioral characteristics of specific groups of patients such as those with low back pain, fibrocitis, headache, and so on. For the reader who desires more information about this test, a good reference is Graham (1977).

The California Psychological Inventory (CPI) (Gough, 1975) is a test similar to the MMPI in terms of how items are answered. Here, however, the scales by which the items are interpreted are based on measured characteristics of "normal" populations; that is, the test taker is compared not to a group with a psychiatric diagnosis, but to nondiagnosed groups of people in whom certain behavioral characteristics have been determined. The CPI also includes a scale that reveals whether test-taking attitude is conscientious and honest. Altogether, the CPI has 18 scales, which are basically divided into four groups: (1) the social ascendancy scales; (2) socialization level and social image scales; (3) intellectual stance scales; and (4) conceptual interest scales. Further description of the interpretation and application of these scales is not possible here. It is sufficient to say that the CPI is geared toward "normal" personality assessment and measures a number of dimensions that are directly relevant to various personality theories. In medical settings to date, however, it has not received the widespread usage, and consequent validation, that the MMPI has enjoyed.

The 16 Personality Factor Questionnaire (16PF) (Cattell, Eber, and Tatsuoka, 1970) is another self-report inventory designed to measure personality dimensions—as the name implies, sixteen in all. This test is considerably more sophisticated in the statistical sense than either the MMPI or CPI. However, its use has been limited, primarily because it is not widely accepted as clinically useful. Nevertheless, it does occasionally surface in medical settings, especially those involving research applications.

The Jenkins Activity Survey (JAS) (Jenkins, Zyzanski, and Rosenman, 1979) is a sixty-one item multiple-choice test used to measure characteristics of Type A (coronary prone) behavior. Although it is not widely used clinically, it is commonly employed for research purposes. High scores on this test indicate approximately a doubled risk of new coronary heart disease as compared to the risk associated with low scores.

The Internal-External Locus of Control Scale (I-E Scale) (Rotter, Seeman, and Liverant, 1962) and the Repression-Sensitization Scale (Byrne, 1964) are multiple-choice self-report inventories consisting of items designed to measure characteristics of the dimensions noted in their titles. The items for these scales were intuitively chosen according to their assumed capacity to reflect the personality dimensions in question. The items were later modified according to psychological testing criteria such that they effectively separated groups of subjects along the desired parameters.

Overall, objective tests are popular in health care settings due to their ease of administration (the patients take the test themselves), because their results are easily compared between patients or within the same patient over time, and because the results are easily quantifiable for research applications. The main disadvantage of objective tests is that they do not necessarily give a truly individual picture of the patient, particularly when manipulated by patients who choose only the "good" response to describe themselves.

Projective Tests

In contrast to the objective tests, projective tests involve fixed questions (stimuli) that leave the responses open-ended. The test takers, in this case, are provided with no clue as to whether their answers are correct or incorrect, desirable or undesirable, common or rare. Since every test taker is different, the results of such tests are difficult to compare among individuals or within the same person over time. However, the projective tests do provide a highly individual picture of behavior and thus yield information as to the unique aspects of behavior organization. A person's response on a projective test is basically determined by his or her own personality, not by the limits placed on answers.

Probably the most popular of the projective tests is the *Rorschach* test (Rorschach, 1921), which consists of ten cards, each containing an inkblot. The subject is shown the cards one at a time and asked to give an interpretation of each. The examiner later questions the subject about the characteristics of the cards that led to each perception. The inkblots themselves are not designed to represent anything in particular; what is seen is the result of the subject's own interpretations. The subject's responses are scored according to standard criteria (Beck, Beck, Levitt, and Molish, 1961), and personality assessments are made on the basis of how and why the subject saw what was reported and what was said about each perception.

Of course, the reliability of this test (that is, its capacity to elicit the same responses each time it is administered) is precluded by the ambiguity of the stimuli. However, most clinical psychologists who use it feel that its lack of reliability reflects its accuracy in capturing the shifting nuances of personal style rather than an inaccurate portrayal of behavioral characteristics. Indeed, only a test such as the Rorschach could detect the various pecularities of thought and perception easily avoided in a more structured situation, such as an objective test, which permits the subject to choose among the alternatives given. There is considerable literature supporting the use of the Rorschach (as well as literature not quite so favorable).

The Thematic Apperception Test (TAT) (Murray, 1943) consists of twenty pictures of people and objects in which the portrayals are rather ambiguous. Here, the subject is asked to tell a story about each picture, with descriptions of what is happening, what the people are thinking and feeling, what led up to the scene, and how it is going to end. The stories created reveal much about the subject's interpersonal relationships, feelings or mood states, issues of concern, probabilities of certain behaviors, and so on. The TAT is also commonly used in medical settings, especially those situations in which particular aspects of interpersonal behavior are of interest.

The third major type of projective test involves the use of incomplete sentences. Here, a number of sentence stems are provided, which a subject is asked to complete (e.g., I secretly _____.). These tests take several forms, some of the most popular being those

101

of Rotter (1950). Incomplete sentence tests are designed for use with different age groups, that is, with children, high-school students, adults, and college students. Basically, their purpose is to provide an indication of what the subject is thinking about at the time the test is being taken. Scoring methods are also available for these tests that permit placement of responses into particular categories. Incomplete sentence tests are popular in medical settings because of their general ease of administration (the patients take these tests themselves) and because they provide straightforward indications about patients' personal concerns, needs, conflicts, desired rewards, and so on.

The last major group of projective tests commonly used in medical settings are projective drawings. For this test, subjects are given a blank piece of paper and asked to draw something. Examples of these tests are the House-Tree-Person test (HTP) (Buck, 1948), with revised scoring systems (Bieliauskas, 1981), and the Draw-A-Person test (Goodenough, 1926). By means of projective drawing tests, an examiner can make inferences about the personality structure of the subject based on the manner in which the drawing is made. As with the Rorschach and TAT tests, the unconstricted responses of the test takers are determined by their own perceptions and understandings. These responses, in the form of drawings, are scored according to size, style, detailing, and other criteria. Observations and research over long periods of time have revealed certain patterns in these drawings, which have then been correlated with specific patterns of personality organization.

BEHAVIORAL ASSESSMENT

Behavioral assessment involves the direct measurement of particular behaviors and the variables that control them, as opposed to the other indirect methods we have discussed. Interviewing, objective testing, and projective testing all make inferences about behaviors based on certain information. Behavioral assessment makes no inferences; rather, it directly measures the behavior in question. If, for example, we wish to determine the likelihood that someone will get out of bed at 7:00 A.M., we will directly measure the action itself and what conditions influenced it rather than assessing the characteristics of "early risers." Almost by its very definition, behavioral assessment is based on learning approaches to behavior organization. Thus, the elements to be measured are the behavior itself, the preceding stimulus, and the subsequent consequence.

Nelson and Barlow (1981, p. 15) described the primary goals of behavioral assessment as "identification and classification of the target behavior or problem, determination of the organismic and environmental controlling variables, design of a treatment program, and evaluation of the success of this program." The target behavior is the behavior we wish to change. The first step is thus to identify the behavior as well as the group of behaviors it may belong to. For example, if excessive alcohol intake is defined as the target behavior, we must identify the kind of alcohol, how many drinks are taken over what period of time, and the type of behavior it represents to the individual (e.g., social, depressive, or relaxing).

Determination of the organismic and environmental controlling variables basically requires that we specify what makes the behavior happen. Using learning principles, we can identify the conditioned stimulus or stimuli, reinforcements, and cue-producing responses. In the case of the problem drinker, a stimulus might be watching television after dinner; the reinforcement might be a feeling of relaxation; and the cue-producing responses might be finishing dinner, which leads to turning on the television, which leads to sitting down in a particular chair, which leads to getting up and making a drink.

The design of a treatment program may also involve learning principles such as the concept of extinction or the process by which inappropriate behaviors are replaced. Referring again to our example, the problem drinker might be forbidden to watch television, thus breaking the sequence of cue-producing responses that lead to eventual reinforcement of the undesirable behavior.

Finally, the success of the treatment program must be evaluated. Since the behavior was initially measured, we can measure it again to see if it has changed. Given our definition of the target behavior in the example above, we may wish to see if the frequency of alcohol consumption has changed. If it hasn't, another treatment program must be initiated. Generally, follow-up evaluations, at time intervals such as three months, six months, or one year, are required to ensure that the changes in behavior are maintained. It is precisely this evaluation of the changes in target behaviors that accounts for the appeal of behavioral assessment: the assessments can be verified, replicated, and/or disproved.

APPLICATIONS IN HEALTH AND ILLNESS

Beyond the preliminary interview, the nature of the information to be obtained in subsequent detailed interviews, psychological tests, and behavioral assessments is such that specific training in the procedures and their interpretation is required. Therefore, when subtle and/or complex information about personality or behavioral organization is needed in the treatment of a patient, consultation with a mental health professional is recommended. Such personality assessment can provide important information as to what the symptoms mean for the patient; how the patient is likely to react to them; whether or not aspects of personality contribute to symptom presentation, formation, or exacerbation; and how the patient is likely to react to the course of illness and the treatment provided.

Let us now look at several examples of personality assessment as they relate to various issues concerning illness and health. Pancheri et al. (1978) examined male subjects admitted to an intensive coronary care unit following severe heart attack. Using the MMPI, they found overall elevations on the clinical scales of this test to be related to poorer clinical condition (i.e., lack of improvement) seven to ten days following admission (see Figure 9). Another study conducted by Leavitt and Garron (1982) used the Rorschach test to examine patients with low back pain. They found that the Rorschach revealed specific characteristics associated with a lack of demonstated physical basis for the pain and that this information expanded on the data for the same patient provided by the MMPI. A final example is provided by Redd (1980), who used behavioral assessment as a means of devising treatment for symptoms of cough and regurgitation of saliva in patients who were receiving chemotherapy for acute leukemia. I cite these examples only to give a sense of the wide range of applications of personality assessment in health care. The specific reports are far too numerous to be described here, but comprehensive coverage of the current areas of related research can be found in the following journals: *General Hospital Psychiatry, Health Psychology, Journal of Behavioral Medicine, Journal of Consulting and*

FIGURE 9. MMPI mean profiles for "improved" and "not-improved" patients after heart attack. (From Pancheri et al., 1978, Figure 1, p. 21. Reprinted by permission of the *Journal of Human Stress* and the author.)

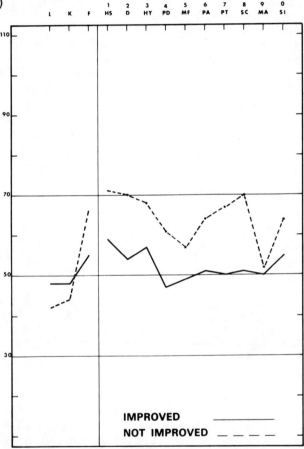

Clinical Psychology, Psychological Medicine, and *Psychosomatic Medicine.* The specific predictors of behavioral characteristics associated with prognosis, maintenance of medical regimen, and patient comfort in particular illnesses are among the many topics you will find of interest.

AN ECLECTIC APPROACH TOWARD INDIVIDUAL DIFFERENCES

In this volume, I have attempted to delineate some of the many different ways in which we can view the organization of behavior. Each viewpoint is complex in and of itself, but it is not likely that any one is entirely correct to the exclusion of the others. Given such diversity in the conceptualizations of personality and granting that much of it is well-founded, it is suggested that the reader keep an open mind in adopting any theory of personality as an aid to understanding the behavior of individual patients.

Close attention to the unconscious factors in patient behavior frequently provides a clear understanding of that behavior. Though less popular today, such an approach frequently provides important information about a patient's symptoms.

Equally effective under different circumstances, perhaps, are the approaches of learning theory and their applications to health care. More readily than with unconscious factors, the health care professional can focus directly on undesirable behaviors and on the situations controlling them, after which implementation of effective strategies to alter those behaviors can be devised. As mentioned in previous chapters, such behaviors can range from vomiting to heart rate to compliance with medical regimens.

The practical application of personality theory to health care problems is generally neither as theoretically complicated as the analytic approaches nor as straightforward and brief as learning theory approaches would boast. Often, the other theories—the interpersonal and cognitive approaches—describe the steady, longer, and more permanent changes we see in behavior. When one can apply the knowledge in such approaches, combined with the techniques of other approaches, intervention can change the "fictions" or "constructs" or "expectancies" that govern how a stimulus is perceived or an impulse is translated. Unfortunately, in the immediate health care situation, the longer approaches are impractical for intervention even though they may help our understanding. When necessary, referrals can be made to mental health professionals to work with patients in this regard.

Overall, the complexity of personality theories is minimal compared to the differences between the individuals they are designed to describe. It is the frequent failure to predict behavior that has led to the generation of so many theories, none of which, even now, can be considered completely predictive or comprehensive. We are thus left with the question of how to choose between them. It is not uncommon to adopt an *eclectic* approach when faced with the individual patient. An eclectic approach "involves the selective application of basic science methods using the most valid current knowledge available for specific clinical situations according to indications and contraindications. It is not committed to any parochial theory of Man" (Thorne, 1973, p. 445). In other words, the eclectic approach selects those aspects of the available theories that are most appropriate for understanding the behavior of a particular individual. Indeed, it would not be at all unreasonable to view a patient from a perspective such as this one:

> A young, single patient with a professional occupation is hospitalized with pneumonia. The patient is extraordinarily difficult to manage because he antagonizes the health care personnel by making demands on them; he also refuses to cooperate with treatment and is very emotional. When the patient's parents visit, all appears to be peaceful; but following each visit, his behavioral difficulties become much more pronounced. Overall, the patient's behaviors interfere with effective medical treatment.
>
> Careful assessment of the patient yields the picture of a young man who has always been dominated by his parents. The domination extends back to childhood, and the patient recalls only an unhappy life. The patient is an orderly, controlling person, an individual who would be seen, from an analytic point of view, as having a conflict in the anal stage. Hostility seems to be the predominant impulse underlying his behavior,

an impulse that appears to be triggered whenever demands are placed on him. This effect can be interpreted as the patient's reaction to the perception of being controlled. However, the patient also places demands on the staff; specifically, he wants to be placed in a dependent position in some way. Thus, the patient can be viewed analytically as having strong dependent needs, unfulfilled but conflicting with the fear of being controlled.

From an interpersonal standpoint, the patient sees the world as wanting to control him and also as failing to meet his needs. The conflict persists. Most likely labeled as a "difficult child" in earlier life, he continues to live up to the expectations imposed by this label. Perceiving his significant others (parents) as cold and rejecting, the patient anticipates such treatment from people in general. His attempts to control interpersonal situations are thus fraught with anger and cause many difficulties.

From a behavioral standpoint, the patient's conflict can be described as one of approach-avoidance with others, including medical staff. He may approach people with a need for dependency and closeness, but as he gets closer, behaviors occur that push them off. Although closeness and dependency are desired by the patient, they are also associated with vulnerability to rejection. On the other hand, expressions of respect or recognition of the patient's professional status are rewarding and make the patient happier.

From a cognitive standpoint, the patient's feelings of rejection can be seen as tied to the label of "difficult child," which by now has been formed by the patient into a construct of general incompetence or failure to achieve. He does have a professional occupation, but somehow this status is not deserved. Thus, his expectancy of failure is high.

The patient has a generally high internal locus of control. He is also highly intelligent and clearly understands the medical situation he is in. Interviews with the patient reveal a sharp sensitivity to being patronized or not having things explained to him.

The information supplied thus far yields some idea of the patient's personality and of certain possible avenues of approach. We might first attend to the patient's conflict as well as to those behaviors that appear to make him feel more satisfied. Treating him with respect and recognizing his professional status, and tying this respect to acceptable patient behaviors, may be a start in the right direction. Although the patient appears to be quite dependent, fulfillment of the demands related to this need might be threatening; thus, we might meet some of his demands, but without becoming too familiar. We might also make sure that the patient is not treated in a way reminiscent of his relationship with his parents; rather, he should be regarded as a peer or colleague in an attempt to maximize the discrepancy between the patient's expectations or perceptions and the real situation. We might also leave the patient alone for a while following his parents' visits, or ask him if he would like to shorten their visits (i.e., "have more privacy").

Many different approaches are included in this perspective, none of which is exclusive of the others. These approaches have been integrated into a whole that provides the most efficient clues to understanding and dealing with this particular patient.

One final point to be made is that patients are not alone in having individual differences; health professionals do, as well. Many of the characteristics discussed throughout this volume describe behaviors you have probably noticed in yourself. Thus, it is important to remember that health professionals react to patients and their behaviors with similar sets of impulses, conflicts, stimulus and response patterns, expectancies, and styles as the patients draw upon in reacting to their symptoms and the settings designed for their care. The interaction between the health professional and the patient will certainly be influenced by personality factors on both sides, which in themselves can be viewed from the variety of approaches discussed.

An appreciation of individual differences among patients, and between all others and ourselves, provides a rich, stimulating, and effective experience in the promotion of health and the treatment of illness. It also prevents us from making generalizations that may be neither appropriate to nor beneficial for the individual patient. In short, close attention to the individual personality will be amply rewarded by positive individual behaviors and successful medical outcomes in the health care setting.

BIBLIOGRAPHY

Achterberg, J., Kenner, C., and Lawlis, F. Biofeedback imagery/desensitization, and relaxation: Pain and stress intervention for severely burned patients. Paper presented at the meeting of the Biofeedback Society of America, Chicago, 1982.

Ackerman, S.H., Manaker, S., and Cohen, J.I. Recent separation and the onset of peptic ulcer disease in older children and adolescents. *Psychosomatic medicine,* 1981, *43,* 305–310.

Adler, A. *The education of children.* London: George Allen & Unwin, 1930.

_____. *Understanding human nature.* New York: Fawcett World Library, 1954.

_____. *The problems of neurosis.* New York: Harper & Row, 1964.

_____. *The practice and theory of individual psychology.* New York: Humanities Press, 1968.

Alexander, F. *Psychosomatic medicine.* New York: Norton, 1950.

Allport, G.W. *Personality: A psychological interpretation.* New York: Holt, 1937.

_____. *Pattern and growth in personality.* New York: Holt, Rinehart, & Winston, 1961.

_____. The general and the unique in psychological science. *Journal of personality,* 1962, *30,* 405–422.

Ansbacher, H.L. and Ansbacher, R.R. (Eds.) *The individual psychology of Alfred Adler.* New York: Basic Books, 1956.

Bakal, D.A. *Psychology and medicine.* New York: Springer, 1979.

Bandura, A. *Principles of behavior modification.* New York: Holt, Rinehart, & Winston, 1969.

Beck, S.J., Beck, A.G., Levitt, E.E., and Molish, H.B. *Rorschach's test I. Basic processes.* New York: Grune & Stratton, 1961.

Belar, C.D. A comment on Silver and Blanchard's (1978) review of the treatment of tension headaches in EMG feedback and relaxation training. *Journal of behavioral medicine,* 1978, *2,* 215–220.

Bieliauskas, L.A. *Stress and its relationship to health and illness*. Boulder, Colorado: Westview Press, 1982.

Bieliauskas, V.J. *Cognitive style scoring system for H-T-P drawings*. Cincinnati, Ohio: Xavier University Press, 1981.

Billingham, K.A. *Developmental psychology for the health care professions, Part 1. Prenatal through adolescent development*. Boulder, Colorado: Westview Press, 1982.

Binet, A. and Simon, T. *A method of measuring the development of the intelligence of young children*. Translated by Clara H. Town. Chicago: Chicago Medical Book Co., 1915.

Buck, J. H-T-P technique: A qualitative and quantitative scoring manual. *Journal of clinical psychology* (Monograph Supplement No. 5), 1948.

Byrne, D. Repression-sensitization as a dimension of personality. In B.A. Maher (Ed.) *Progress in experimental personality research, Vol. 1*. New York: Academic Press, 1964.

Cattell, R.B., Eber, H.W., and Tatsuoka, M.M. *Handbook for the sixteen personality factor questionnaire*. Champaign, Illinois: Institute for Personality and Ability Testing, 1970.

Cohen, J.J., McArthur, D.L. and Rickles, W.H. Comparison of four biofeedback treatments for migraine headache: Physiological and headache variables. *Psychosomatic medicine*, 1980, *42*, 463–480.

Counte, M.A. and Christman, L.P. *Interpersonal behavior and health care*. Boulder, Colorado: Westview Press, 1981.

Cromwell, R.L., Butterfield, E.C., Brayfield, F.M., and Curry, J.J. *Acute myocardial infarction: Reaction and recovery*. St. Louis: Mosby, 1977.

Dollard, J. and Miller, N.E. *Personality and psychotherapy: An analysis in terms of learning, thinking, and culture*. New York: McGraw-Hill, 1950.

Downie, N.M. and Heath, R.W. *Basic statistical methods*. New York: Harper & Row, 1965.

Dunbar, H.F. *Psychosomatic diagnosis*. New York: Hoeber, 1943.

Dunn, L.M. *Peabody picture vocabulary test*. Circle Pines, Minnesota: American Guidance Service, 1959.

Dunn, L.M. and Markwardt, F.L. *PIAT: Peabody individual achievement test*. Circle Pines, Minnesota: American Guidance Service, 1970.

Egbert, L., Battit, G., Welch, C., and Bartlett, M. Reduction of postoperative pain by encouragement and instruction of patients. *New England journal of medicine*, 1964, *270*, 825–827.

Epstein, S. and Fenz, W.D. The detection of areas of emotional stress through variations in perceptual threshold and physiological arousal. *Journal of experimental research and personality*, 1967, *3*, 191–199.

Eysenck, H.J. Extraversion and the acquisition of eyeblink and GSR conditioned responses. *Psychological bulletin*, 1965, *63*, 258–270.

Ferster, C.B. and Skinner, B.F. *Schedules of reinforcement.* New York: Appleton-Century-Crofts, 1957.

Fordyce, W.E. *Behavioral methods for chronic pain and illness.* St. Louis: Mosby, 1976.

Freud, S. *The standard edition of the complete psychological works of Sigmund Freud. Vols. I–XXIII.* London: Hogarth Press, 1953–1964.

_____. *Totem and taboo and other works. Vol. XIII. The standard edition of the complete psychological works of Sigmund Freud.* London: Hogarth Press, 1955.

_____. *The ego and the id and other works. Vol. XIX. The standard edition of the complete psychological works of Sigmund Freud.* London: Hogarth Press, 1961.

Friedman, M. and Rosenman, R.H. *Type A behavior and your heart.* New York: Knopf, 1974.

Gentry, W.D. Noncompliance to medical regimen. In R.B. Williams and W.D. Gentry (Eds.) *Behavioral approaches to medical treatment.* Cambridge, Massachusetts: Ballinger, 1977.

Getzels, J.W. and Jackson, P.W. The study of giftedness: A multidimensional approach. In L.E. Tyler (Ed.) *Intelligence: Some recurring issues.* New York: Van Nostrand, 1969.

Glass, D.C. Stress, behavior patterns, and coronary disease. *American scientist,* 1977, *65,* 177–187.

Goodenough, F.C. *Measurement of intelligence by drawings.* New York: World Book Co., 1926.

Gordon, J.E. Interpersonal prediction of repressors and sensitizers. *Journal of personality,* 1957, *25,* 686–698.

Gordon, L.B. *Behavioral intervention in health care.* Boulder, Colorado: Westview Press, 1981.

Gough, H.G. *Manual for the California psychological inventory.* Palo Alto, California: Consulting Psychologists Press, 1975.

Graham, J.R. *The MMPI: A practical guide.* New York: Oxford, 1977.

Guilford, J.P. Three faces of intellect. *American psychologist,* 1959, *14,* 469–479.

Hall, C.S. and Lindzey, G. *Theories of personality.* New York: Wiley, 1970.

Hamilton, M. Development of a rating scale for primary depressive illness. *British journal of social and clinical psychology,* 1967, *6,* 278–296.

Hathaway, S.R. and McKinley, J.C. *The Minnesota multiphasic personality inventory manual.* New York: Psychological Corporation, 1943.

Hilgard, E.R. *Theories of learning.* New York: Appleton-Century-Crofts, 1956.

Hull, C.L. *A behavior system.* New Haven, Connecticut: Yale University Press, 1952.

Humphreys, L.G. The organization of human abilities. *American psychologist,* 1962, *17,* 475–483.

Janis, I.L. *Psychological stress.* New York: Wiley, 1958.

Jastak, J.F. and Jastak, S.R. *WRAT Manual. The wide range achievement test.* Wilmington, Delaware: Guidance Association of Delaware, Inc., 1965.

Jenkins, C.D., Zyzanski, S.J., and Rosenman, R.H. *Manual for the Jenkins activity survey.* New York: Psychological Corporation, 1979.

Jung, C.G. *Psychological types.* New York: Harcourt, Brace & World, 1923.

———. *The collected works of C.G. Jung. Vols. 1–17.* H. Read, M. Fordham, and G. Adler (Eds.), Bollingen Series. New York: Pantheon Books, 1953–1971.

Kahn, T.C. and Giffen, M.D. *Psychological techniques in diagnosis and evaluation.* New York: Pergamon, 1960.

Kelly, G.A. *The psychology of personal constructs. Volume one: A theory of personality.* New York: Norton, 1955a.

———. *The psychology of personal constructs. Volume two: Clinical diagnosis and psychotherapy.* New York: Norton, 1955b.

Klepac, R.K., McDonald, M., Hauge, G., and Dowling, J. Reactions to pain among subjects high and low in dental fear. *Journal of behavioral medicine,* 1980, *3,* 373–384.

Kobasa, S. Stressful life events, personality, and health: An inquiry into hardiness. *Journal of personality and social psychology,* 1979, *37,* 1–11.

Korchin, S.J. *Modern clinical psychology.* New York: Basic Books, 1976.

Krech, D. and Crutchfield, R.S. *Elements of psychology.* New York: Knopf, 1965.

Lang, P.J. and Melamed, B.G. Case report: Avoidance conditioning therapy of an infant with chronic ruminative vomiting. *Journal of abnormal psychology,* 1969, *74,* 1–8.

Leavitt, G. and Garron, D.C. Rorschach and pain characteristics of patients with low back pain and "conversion V" MMPI profiles. *Journal of personality assessment,* 1982, *46,* 18–25.

Lefcourt, H.M. The function of the illusion of control and freedom. *American psychologist,* 1973, *28,* 417–425.

Levy, L.H. *Conceptions of personality: Theories and research.* New York: Random House, 1970.

Lezak, M.D. *Neuropsychological assessment.* New York: Oxford, 1976.

London, J. *The call of the wild.* New York: New American Library, 1960.

Lopez, M.A. and Feldman, H. *Developmental psychology for the health care professions: Part 2—Adulthood and aging.* Boulder, Colorado: Westview Press, 1982.

Lorr, M.L., McNair, D.M., Klett, C.J., and Lasky, J.J. *Inpatient multidimensional psychiatric scale (IMPS).* Palo Alto, California: Consulting Psychologists Press, 1966.

McNemar, Q. Lost: Our intelligence? Why? *American psychologist,* 1964, *19,* 871–882.

Matarazzo, J.D. *Wechsler's measurement and appraisal of adult intelligence.* Baltimore: Williams & Wilkins, 1972.

Matteson, M.H. and Ivancevich, J.M. The coronary-prone behavior pattern: A review and appraisal. *Social science and medicine,* 1980, *14A,* 337–351.

Melamed, B.G. and Seigel, L. Reduction of anxiety in children facing hospital-ization and surgery by use of filmed modeling. *Journal of consulting and clinical psychology,* 1975, *43,* 511–521.

_____. *Behavioral medicine: Practical applications in health care.* New York: Springer, 1980.

Mikulic, M.A. Reinforcement of independent and dependent patient be-haviors by nursing personnel: An exploratory study. *Nursing research,* 1971, *20,* 162–165.

Miller, N.E. Experimental studies of conflict. In J. McVicker Hunt (Ed.) *Person-ality and the behavioral disorders. Vol. I.* New York: Ronald, 1944.

Montgomery, G.K. and Cleeland, C.S. Management of Parkinsonian symp-toms by multimodal behavior therapy. Paper presented at the meeting of the American Psychological Association, Montreal, 1980.

Morgan, C.T. and King, R.A. *Introduction to psychology.* New York: McGraw-Hill, 1971.

Mowrer, O.H. A stimulus-response analysis of anxiety and its role as a rein-forcing agent. *Psychological review,* 1939, *46,* 553–566.

Murray, E.J. and Jacobsen, L.A. The nature of learning in traditional and be-havioral psychotherapy. In A.E. Bergin and S.L. Garfield (Eds.) *Handbook of psychotherapy and behavior change.* New York: Wiley, 1971.

Murray, H. *Thematic apperception test.* Cambridge, Massachusetts: Harvard University Press, 1943.

Nelson, R.O. and Barlow, D.H. Behavioral assessment: Basic strategies and initial procedures. In D.H. Barlow (Ed.) *Behavioral assessment of adult disorders.* New York: Guilford, 1981.

Orth-Gomer, K., Ahlborn, A., and Theorell, T. Impact of pattern A behavior on ischemic heart disease when controlling for conventional risk in-dicators. *Journal of human stress,* 1980, *6,* 6–13.

Pancheri, P., Bellaterra, M., Matteoli, S., Cristofari, M., Polizzi, C., and Puletti, M. Infarct as a stress agent: Life history and personality characteristics in improved versus not-improved patients after severe heart attack. *Journal of human stress,* 1978, *4,* 16–22, 41–42.

Pavlov, I.P. *Conditioned reflexes: An investigation of the physiological activity of the cerebral cortex.* New York: Oxford, 1927.

Petrie, A. *Individuality in pain and suffering.* Chicago: University of Chicago Press, 1967.

Psychology today: An introduction. Del Mar, California: CRM Books, 1972.

Redd, W.H. Stimulus control and extinction of psychosomatic symptoms in cancer patients in protective isolation. *Journal of consulting and clinical psychology*, 1980, *48*, 448–455.

Redd, W.H., Andreasen, G.V., and Minagawa, R.Y. Hypnotic control of anticipatory emesis in patients receiving cancer chemotherapy. *Journal of consulting and clinical psychology*, 1982, *50*, 14–19.

Rorschach, H. *Psychodiagnostics*. New York: Grune & Stratton, 1921.

Rosenman, R.H. The interview method of assessment of the coronary prone behavior pattern. In J.M. Dembroski, S.M. Weiss, J.L. Shields, S.G. Haynes, and M. Feinleib (Eds.) *Coronary prone behavior*. New York: Springer-Verlag, 1978.

Rosenman, R.H., Brand, R.J. Jenkins, C.D., Friedman, M., Straus, R., and Wurm, M. Coronary heart disease in the Western Collaborative Group Study: Final follow-up experience of 8½ years. *Journal of the American Medical Association*, 1975, *233*, 872–877.

Roskies, E., Kearny, H., Spevack, M., Surkis, A., Cohen, C., and Gilman, S. Generalization and durability of treatment efforts in an intervention program for coronary-prone (Type A) managers. *Journal of behavioral medicine*, 1979, *2*, 195–207.

Roskies, E., Spevack, M., Surkis, A., Cohen, C., and Gilman, S. Changing the coronary-prone (Type A) behavior pattern in a nonclinical population. *Journal of behavioral medicine*, 1978, *1*, 210–216.

Rotter, J.B. *Incomplete sentences blank*. New York: Psychological Corporation, 1950.

_____. *Social learning and clinical psychology*. Englewood Cliffs, New Jersey: Prentice-Hall, 1954.

Rotter, J.B., Chance, J.E., and Phares, E.J. *Applications of a social learning theory of personality*. New York: Holt, Rinehart & Winston, 1972.

Rotter, J.B., Seeman, M., and Liverant, S. Internal vs. external locus of control of reinforcement: A major variable in behavior therapy. In N.F. Washburne (Ed.) *Decisions, values, and groups*. London: Pergamon, 1962.

Rychlak, J.F. *Introduction to personality and psychotherapy*. Boston: Houghton Mifflin, 1973, 1981.

Schacter, S. and Singer, J.E. Cognitive, social, and physiological determinants of emotional state. *Psychological review*, 1962, *69*, 379–399.

Schwartz, G.E. and Beatty, J. *Biofeedback theory and research*. New York: Academic Press, 1977.

Shipley, R.H., Butt, J.H., and Horowitz, E.A. Preparation to reexperience a stressful medical examination: Effects of repetitious videotape exposure and coping style. *Journal of consulting and clinical psychology*, 1979, *47*, 485–499.

Silver, B.V. and Blanchard, E.G. Biofeedback and relaxation training in the treatment of psychophysiological disorders: Or, are the machines really necessary? *Journal of behavioral medicine,* 1978, *1,* 217–239.

Skinner, B.F. *The behavior of organisms—An experimental analysis.* New York: Appleton-Century, 1938.

Sloan, W. and Birch, J.W. A rationale for degrees of retardation. *American journal of mental deficiency,* 1955, *60,* 262.

Spearman, C. *The abilities of man.* New York: Macmillan, 1927.

Spearman, C. and Jones W. *Human abilities.* London: Macmillan, 1950.

Spence, K.W. Cognitive and drive factors in the extinction of the conditional eye blink in human subjects. *Psychological review,* 1966, *73,* 445–458.

Spitzer, R.L. and Endicott, J. *Schedule for affective disorders and schizophrenia: SADS.* Bethesda, Maryland: National Institute of Mental Health, 1978.

Stern, W.L. The psychological methods of testing intelligence. Translated by G.M. Whipple. *Educational psychology monographs,* No. 13. Baltimore: Warwick & York, 1914.

Sternbach, R.A. *Pain patients: traits and treatment.* New York: Academic Press, 1974.

Strain, J.J. and Grossman, S. *Psychological care of the medically ill.* New York: Appleton-Century-Crofts, 1975.

Suinn, R.M. Behavior therapy for cardiac patients. *Behavior therapy,* 1974, *5,* 569–571.

_____. Type A behavior pattern. In R.B. Williams and W.D. Gentry (Eds.) *Behavioral approaches to medical treatment.* Cambridge, Massachusetts: Ballinger, 1977.

Sullivan, H.S. *The interpersonal theory of psychiatry.* New York: Norton, 1953.

_____. *The fusion of psychiatry and social science.* New York: Norton, 1964.

Terman, L.M. *The measurement of intelligence.* Boston: Houghton Mifflin, 1916.

Terman, L.M. and Merrill, M.A. *The Stanford-Binet intelligence scale* (1972 norms edition). Boston: Houghton Mifflin, 1973.

Thorne, F.C. Eclectic psychotherapy. In R. Corsin (Ed.) *Current psychotherapies.* Itasca, Illinois: F.E. Peacock, 1973.

Vaihinger, H. *The philosophy of "as if."* New York: Harcourt, Brace & World, 1925.

Wechsler, D. *WPPSI manual. Wechsler preschool and primary scale of intelligence.* New York: Psychological Corporation, 1967.

_____. *WISC-R manual. Wechsler intelligence scale for children—revised.* New York: Psychological Corporation, 1974.

_____. *WAIS-R manual. Wechsler adult intelligence scale—revised.* New York: Psychological Corporation, 1981.

Weiner, H. *Psychobiology and human disease.* New York: Elsevier, 1977.

Weiner, H., Thaler, M., Reiser, M.F., and Mirsky, A. Etiology of duodenal ulcer. I. Relation of specific psychological characteristics to rate of gastric secretion (serum pepsinogen). *Psychosomatic medicine*, 1957, *19*, 1–10.

Weinman, J. *An outline of psychology as applied to medicine*. Bristol, England: John Wright & Sons, 1981.

Williams, R.B. and Gentry, W.D. (Eds.) *Behavioral approaches to medical treatment*. Cambridge, Massachusetts: Ballinger, 1977.

Ziegler, F.J., Imboden, J.B., and Meyer, E. Contemporary conversion reactions: A clinical study. *American journal of psychiatry*, 1960, *116*, 901–910.

INDEX

defined, 3–4
independent concepts of, 71–78
interpersonal approach, 107,
109. See also Adler, Alfred;
Sullivan, Harry Stack
normal, 99
psychoanalytic theory of. See
Psychoanalysis
sex-typing of, 48
and world view, 4–5
See also Dynamic perspective;
Heart disease, and Type A
personality; Individual
behavior
Personifications, 29
Pessimist, 27
Petrie, A., 71, 72
Phallic stage, 9, 10, 11
Phares, E. J., 66
PIAT. See Peabody Individual
Achievement Test
Pleasure principle, 8, 9, 10, 11,
18, 46
Pre-adolescence stage, 31
Preconscious, 11(fig.), 12, 13
Primary function. See Superior
function
Projection, 14
Projective tests, 100–102
Prototaxic experience, 29–30, 31
Prototypes, 24, 29
Psyche, 15(fig.), 17–18
Psychoanalysis, 8–14
Psychological Medicine, 105
Psychological testing, 93, 97–102
Psychosomatic Medicine, 105
Puberty, 10
Punishment, 49, 59

Rating scales, 96
Rational functions. See Feeling;
Thinking

Reaction formation, 14
Realistic anxiety, 13
Reality, approaches to, 27
Reality principle, 12
Redd, W. H., 104
Reducer, 71, 72, 78
Reflected appraisals, 28, 64
Regional enteritis, 19
Reinforcement, 40, 43, 46, 49–51,
52(fig.), 58–59, 64, 103
values (RV), 65–66
Reiser, M. F., 20
Relaxation, 57, 59
Repression, 11(fig.), 12, 13, 14,
25, 30, 46–47, 75, 98
-sensitization, 75–76, 100
Respondent behavior, 38. See also
Operant conditioning
Response, 38, 39, 41–42, 46–47
non-verbal, 41, 46–47, 48
See also Language
Rewards, 50
Rheumatoid arthritis, 19
Role formation, 63
Rorschach test, 101, 102, 104
Rosenman, R. H., 76
Rotter, Julian B., 61, 62, 64–66,
67, 102
Ruling approach, 27
RV. See Reinforcement, values
Rychlak, J. F., 24, 39

SADS. See Schedule for Affective
Disorders and Schizophrenia
Salutogenic cure, 73, 74
Schacter, S., 58
Schedule for Affective Disorders
and Schizophrenia (SADS), 96
Schwartz, G. E., 59
Secondary functions, 17, 18(fig.)
Security, 29, 30
Selective inattention, 30